United States General Accounting Office

GAO

Report to the Chairman, Subcommittee on Asia and the Pacific, Committee on International Relations, House of Representatives

April 2004

EMERGING INFECTIOUS DISEASES

Asian SARS Outbreak Challenged International and National Responses

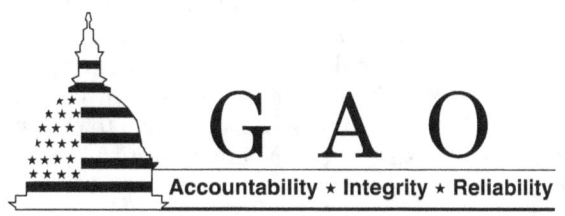

GAO

Accountability ★ Integrity ★ Reliability

GAO-04-564

April 2004

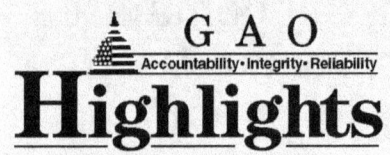

GAO
Accountability • Integrity • Reliability

Highlights

Highlights of GAO-04-564, a report to the Chairman, Subcommittee on Asia and the Pacific, Committee on International Relations, House of Representatives

EMERGING INFECTIOUS DISEASES

Asian SARS Outbreak Challenged International and National Responses

Why GAO Did This Study

Severe acute respiratory syndrome (SARS) emerged in southern China in November 2002 and spread rapidly along international air routes in early 2003. Asian countries had the most cases (7,782) and deaths (729). SARS challenged Asian health care systems, disrupted Asian economies, and tested the effectiveness of the International Health Regulations. GAO was asked to examine the roles of the World Health Organization (WHO), the U.S. government, and Asian governments (China, Hong Kong, and Taiwan) in responding to SARS; the estimated economic impact of SARS in Asia; and efforts to update the International Health Regulations.

What GAO Recommends

GAO is recommending that the Secretaries of Health and Human Services (HHS) and State work with WHO and other member states to strengthen WHO's global infectious disease network. GAO is also recommending that the Secretary of HHS complete steps to ensure that the agency can obtain passenger contact information in a timely manner, including, if necessary, the promulgation of specific regulations; and that the Secretary of State work with other relevant agencies to develop procedures for arranging medical evacuations during an airborne infectious disease outbreak. HHS, State, and WHO generally concurred with the report's content and its recommendations.

www.gao.gov/cgi-bin/getrpt?GAO-04-564.

To view the full product, including the scope and methodology, click on the link above. For more information, contact David Gootnick at (202) 512-3149 or Janet Heinrich at (202) 512-7119.

What GAO Found

WHO implemented extensive actions to respond to SARS, but its response was delayed by an initial lack of cooperation from officials in China and challenged by limited resources for infectious disease control. WHO activated its global infectious disease network and deployed public health specialists to affected areas in Asia to provide technical assistance. WHO also established international teams to identify the cause of SARS and provide guidance for managing the outbreak. WHO's ability to respond to SARS in Asia was limited by its authority under the current International Health Regulations and dependent on cooperation from affected areas.

U.S. government agencies played key roles in responding to SARS in Asia and controlling its spread into the United States, but these efforts revealed limitations. The Centers for Disease Control and Prevention supplied public health experts to WHO for deployment to Asia and gave direct assistance to Taiwan. It also tried to contact passengers from flights and ships on which a traveler was diagnosed with SARS after arriving in the United States. However, these efforts were hampered by airline concerns and procedural issues. The State Department helped facilitate the U.S. government's response to SARS but encountered multiple difficulties when it tried to arrange medical evacuations for U.S. citizens infected with SARS overseas.

Although the Asian governments we studied initially struggled to recognize the SARS emergency and organize an appropriate response, they ultimately established control. As the governments have acknowledged, their initial response to SARS was hindered by poor communication, ineffective leadership, inadequate disease surveillance systems, and insufficient public health capacity. Improved screening, rapid isolation of suspected cases, enhanced hospital infection control, and quarantine of close contacts ultimately helped end the outbreak.

The SARS crisis temporarily dampened consumer confidence in Asia, costing Asian economies $11 billion to $18 billion and resulting in estimated losses of 0.5 percent to 2 percent of total output, according to official and academic estimates. SARS had significant, but temporary, negative impacts on a variety of economic activities, especially travel and tourism.

The SARS outbreak added impetus to the revision of the International Health Regulations. WHO and its member states are considering expanding the scope of required disease reporting to include all public health emergencies of international concern and devising a system for better cooperation with WHO and other countries. Some questions are not yet resolved, including WHO's authority to conduct investigations in countries absent their consent, the enforcement mechanism to resolve compliance issues, and how to ensure public health security without unduly interfering with travel and trade.

_____ United States General Accounting Office

Contents

Figures

Abbreviations

CDC	Centers for Disease Control and Prevention
GDP	gross domestic product
GOARN	Global Outbreak Alert and Response Network
GPHIN	Global Public Health Intelligence Network
HHS	Department of Health and Human Services
SARS	severe acute respiratory syndrome
WHO	World Health Organization
WPRO	Western Pacific Regional Office

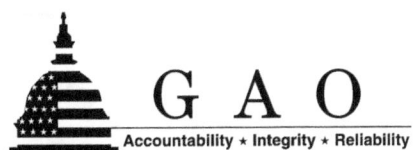

G A O
Accountability ★ Integrity ★ Reliability

United States General Accounting Office
Washington, D.C. 20548

April 28, 2004

The Honorable James A. Leach
Chairman, Subcommittee on Asia
    and the Pacific
Committee on International Relations
House of Representatives

Dear Mr. Chairman:

Severe acute respiratory syndrome (SARS), the first major new infectious disease of the 21st century, emerged in southern China in November 2002. SARS is a contagious respiratory disease with a substantial mortality rate, and there is no vaccine, no reliable rapid diagnostic test, and no specific treatment for the disease. The disease spread rapidly along international air routes through Asia, North America, and Europe in early 2003, eventually infecting 8,098 people and causing 774 deaths.[1] Asian countries were the hardest hit, with 7,782 cases and 729 deaths. The 2002-2003 SARS outbreak presented a challenge to Asian health care systems and disrupted Asian economies. The World Health Organization (WHO), the U.S. government, and Asian governments all played a role in controlling the SARS outbreak in Asia. The history of this effort raises important issues regarding international and national preparedness for recognizing and responding to emerging infectious diseases such as SARS, including the effectiveness of the International Health Regulations, WHO's legal framework for preventing the international spread of infectious diseases.

In light of these concerns, you asked that we assess the impact of SARS on health and commerce in Asia. In this report we examine (1) WHO's actions to respond to the SARS outbreak in Asia, (2) the role of the U.S. government in responding to SARS in Asia and limiting its spread into the United States, (3) how governments in the areas of Asia most affected by SARS responded to the outbreak, (4) the estimated economic impact of SARS in Asia, and (5) the status of efforts to update the International Health Regulations.

---

[1]"Summary of probable SARS cases with onset of illness from 1 November 2002 to 31 July 2003," (Geneva, Switzerland: WHO, September 26, 2003), http://www.who.int/csr/sars/country/table2003_09_23/en/(downloaded March 12, 2004).

The primary focus of our report is on those parts of Asia most severely affected by SARS during the 2002-2003 outbreak, including China, Hong Kong, and Taiwan. To examine the response to the SARS outbreak by WHO, the U.S. government, and Asian governments, we conducted fieldwork in Beijing, Hong Kong and Guangdong Province, China; and in Taipei, Taiwan, where we met with public health officials, including senior Ministry of Health staff, international epidemiologists, and local hospital workers. We supplemented our field-level information with interviews with WHO and U.S. government officials responsible for managing the response to SARS and recognized public health experts; we also reviewed relevant documents and reports. To describe the economic impact of SARS in Asia, we reviewed official macroeconomic and sector data as well as economic impact studies from international financial institutions, industry associations, and public policy research organizations. We determined that the official national accounts data were sufficiently reliable for the purposes of our analysis by reviewing supplementary documentary evidence and each economy's compliance with data dissemination standards. The scope of our summary of economic analyses included other Asian economies strongly impacted by the disease: Malaysia, Singapore, Thailand, and Vietnam. Finally, we examined a draft of WHO's proposed revision of the International Health Regulations and interviewed WHO and U.S. government officials and other legal experts to determine the potential impacts of the revised rules. See pages 46-48 for a more complete description of our scope and methodology. We performed our work from July 2003 to April 2004 in accordance with generally accepted government auditing standards.

Results in Brief

WHO implemented extensive actions to respond to SARS, but its response was delayed by an initial lack of cooperation from officials in China and challenged by limited resources. At the heart of WHO's response to SARS was the activation of its global infectious disease network. This effort, combined with assistance from WHO's Asian regional office, included deploying public health specialists to affected areas in Asia to provide technical assistance and establishing international teams of researchers and clinicians who worked together to identify the cause of SARS, investigate modes of transmission, and develop guidance for managing the outbreak. WHO played a major role in controlling the spread of SARS by issuing global alerts and recommending against travel to countries with SARS outbreaks. It also issued guidance and recommendations to affected areas and the international community on surveillance, preparedness, and response. Although the response was ultimately successful, WHO's actions were delayed because China did not initially provide information about the SARS outbreak or invite WHO to assist in investigating and managing the outbreak in a timely manner. WHO's ability to respond to SARS in China, and elsewhere, was limited by its authority under the current International Health Regulations and dependent on cooperation from affected areas. In addition, WHO's ability to provide timely and appropriate expertise was challenged by the limited resources available to its global infectious disease network, which was stretched to capacity during the outbreak.

U.S. government agencies played significant roles in responding to SARS in Asia and controlling its spread into the United States, but these efforts revealed limitations in their ability to respond to emerging infectious diseases. The Department of Health and Human Services' (HHS) Centers for Disease Control and Prevention (CDC) was involved in early international efforts to identify the disease, provided a significant proportion of the public health experts deployed by WHO to Asia, and gave direct assistance to Taiwanese health authorities. CDC also helped limit the spread of SARS into this country by disseminating information to travelers and attempting to identify and contact passengers from flights and ships on which travelers were diagnosed with SARS after arriving in the United States. However, CDC encountered obstacles that made it unable to perform this important outbreak control measure because of airline concerns over CDC's authority and the privacy of passenger information, as well as procedural issues. CDC is exploring options to overcome the problems it encountered, although it has faced obstacles in pursuing some of them. The State Department (State) applied diplomatic pressure on governments to increase transparency and response, helped facilitate the U.S. government response to SARS in Asia, and provided information on SARS to U.S. government employees and citizens in the region. State also attempted to coordinate medical evacuations for a small number of U.S. citizens infected with SARS overseas but encountered multiple difficulties. These difficulties have not been resolved and could present challenges in the future. Although State has not developed a strategy to address these problems, it is working with other agencies to develop guidance for arranging medical evacuations.

Although the Asian governments we studied initially struggled to recognize the SARS emergency and organize an appropriate response, they ultimately established control. As Asian government officials acknowledged, poor communication, a lack of effective leadership and coordination, and weaknesses in disease surveillance systems and public health capacity constrained their response. In China, poor communication within the country, with Hong Kong and Taiwan, and with WHO obscured the severity of the outbreak during its initial stages. For example, a detailed report produced by provincial officials 2 weeks before China officially announced the SARS outbreak was not shared with other governments or WHO. An initial lack of effective leadership and coordination within the governments of China, Hong Kong, and Taiwan hindered the implementation of a large-scale control effort and led to the dismissal of high-ranking officials. As the outbreak progressed, problems with disease surveillance systems and overall public health capacity further delayed control of the outbreak in many of the affected areas. For example, officials in China noted that a large number of cases in Beijing were not reported because there was no system to collect this information from hospitals in the city. In Taiwan, officials acknowledged that a lack of expertise in hospital infection control contributed to a secondary, and more severe, outbreak in hospitals throughout the island. However, improved screening, rapid isolation of suspected cases, enhanced hospital infection control, and quarantine of close contacts ultimately helped end the outbreak in Asia. In the aftermath of SARS, efforts are under way to improve public health capacity in Asia to better deal with SARS and other infectious disease outbreaks.

The SARS crisis temporarily dampened consumer confidence, costing selected Asian economies around $11 billion to $18 billion and resulting in an estimated loss of 0.5 percent to 2 percent of their total economic output, according to official and academic estimates. Though sectors most affected by SARS have now recovered, the outbreak had a significant negative impact on a variety of economic activities. The most severe economic impacts occurred in the travel and tourism industry, particularly the airline industry. Anecdotal evidence suggests that retail sales, and to a lesser degree some foreign trade and investment, also temporarily declined as a result of SARS. In response to the outbreak, governments in Asia provided economic stimulus packages that also cost billions.

The SARS outbreak added impetus to efforts to revise WHO's International Health Regulations, and an interim draft of revised regulations is currently being circulated. Recognizing that emerging and re-emerging diseases have made the regulations obsolete, WHO and its member states are considering (1) expanding the scope of reporting beyond the three diseases that are currently required to be reported (cholera, plague, and yellow fever) to include all potential public health emergencies of international concern and (2) devising a system for better member state dialogue and cooperation with WHO and other countries. However, important questions about the proposed regulations' scope of coverage, WHO's authority to conduct investigations in countries absent their specific consent, the limited public health capacity of developing countries, the enforcement mechanism used to resolve compliance issues, and how to ensure public health security without unnecessary interference with travel and trade will have to be resolved in the debate leading to the adoption of the final regulations.

We are recommending that the Secretary of Health and Human Services, in collaboration with the Secretary of State, work with WHO and official representatives from other WHO member states to strengthen the response capacity of WHO's global infectious disease network. In light of the unresolved problems of identifying and contacting travelers arriving in the United States who may have been exposed to an infectious disease, and evacuating U.S. government employees overseas who have an airborne infectious disease, we are making two additional recommendations. First, we are recommending that the Secretary of Health and Human Services complete steps to ensure that the agency can obtain passenger contact information in a timely manner, including, if necessary, the promulgation of regulations specifically for this purpose. Second, we are recommending that the Secretary of State work with other relevant agencies to identify public and private sector resources and develop procedures for arranging medical evacuations during an airborne infectious disease outbreak in foreign countries.

In providing written comments on a draft of this report, HHS, State, and WHO generally concurred with the report's content and its recommendations (see apps. IV, V, and VI for a reprint of their comments). They also provided technical and clarifying comments that we have incorporated where appropriate. HHS and State commented that the report provided a good summary of the SARS outbreak and the impact upon and actions taken by affected countries, WHO, and the U.S. government. They endorsed GAO's recommendations but noted that sensitive legal and privacy issues and diplomatic concerns must be carefully addressed in regard to contact tracing of passengers who may have been exposed to an infectious disease. WHO commented that the report provides a factual analysis of the events surrounding the emergence of SARS and the major weaknesses in national and international control efforts. WHO also commented that Asian governments should be better credited for the depth and intensity of their response effort, but we believe the report presents a balanced view. WHO also provided clarifying language on the role of its global response network, which we have incorporated.

Background

SARS is a severe viral infection that is sometimes fatal. The disease first emerged in China in 2002 and then spread through Asia to 26 countries around the world. Although national governments are responsible for responding to infectious disease outbreaks such as SARS, WHO plays an important role in coordinating the response to the global spread of infectious diseases and assisting countries with their public health response to outbreaks. The U.S. government plays a role during international outbreaks in assisting WHO and affected countries and protecting U.S. citizens and interests at home and abroad.

Characteristics of SARS

The virus that causes SARS is a member of a family of viruses known as coronaviruses, which are thought to cause about 10 percent to 15 percent of common colds.[2] Within 2 to 10 days after infection with the SARS virus, an individual may begin to develop symptoms—including cough, fever, and body aches—that are difficult to distinguish from those of other respiratory illnesses. The primary mode of transmission appears to be direct or indirect contact with respiratory secretions or contaminated objects. Another feature of the disease is the occurrence of "superspreading events," where evidence suggests that the disease is transmitted at a high rate due to a combination of patient, environmental, and other factors. According to WHO, the global case fatality rate for SARS is approximately 11 percent and may be more than 50 percent for individuals over age 65.

Prevention and Control of SARS

The management of a SARS outbreak relies on the use of established public health measures for the control of infectious diseases—including case identification and contact tracing, transmission control, and exposure management, defined as follows:

- *Case identification and contact tracing:* defining what symptoms, laboratory results, and medical histories constitute a positive case in a patient and tracing and tracking individuals who may have been exposed to these patients.

---

[2]Scientific evidence suggests that the virus originated in animals and crossed into human populations. See Y. Guan, "Isolation and characterization of viruses related to the SARS coronavirus from animals in southern China," *Science*, vol. 302, no. 5,643 (2003).

- *Transmission control:* controlling the transmission of disease-producing microorganisms through use of proper hand hygiene and personal protective equipment, such as masks, gowns, and gloves.

- *Exposure management:* separating infected and noninfected individuals. Quarantine is a type of exposure management that refers to the separation or restriction of movement of individuals who are not yet ill but were exposed to an infectious agent and are potentially infectious.

The 2002-2003 SARS Outbreak

The emergence of SARS in China can be traced to reports of cases of atypical pneumonia[3] in several cities throughout Guangdong Province in November 2002. (See fig. 1 for a timeline of the emergence of SARS cases and WHO and U.S. government actions.) Because atypical pneumonia is not unusual in this region and the cases did not appear to be connected, many of these early cases were not recognized as a new disease. However, physicians were alarmed because of the unusual number of health care workers who became severely ill after treating patients with a diagnosis of atypical pneumonia. The international outbreak began in February 2003 when an infected physician who had treated some of these patients in China traveled to Hong Kong and stayed at a local hotel. Some individuals who visited the hotel acquired the infection and subsequently traveled to Vietnam, Singapore, and Toronto and seeded secondary outbreaks. Throughout spring 2003, the number of cases continued to spread through Asia to 26 countries around the world, and at its peak—in early May—hundreds of new SARS cases were reported every week. (See app. I for a map of total SARS cases and deaths.) In July 2003, WHO announced that the outbreak had been contained. (See app. II for a detailed chronology of the SARS outbreak.)

---

[3]Atypical pneumonia is caused by a variety of bacteria and viruses and has different clinical signs and a more protracted onset of symptoms compared with other forms of pneumonia.

Figure 1: Timeline of SARS Events and Actions

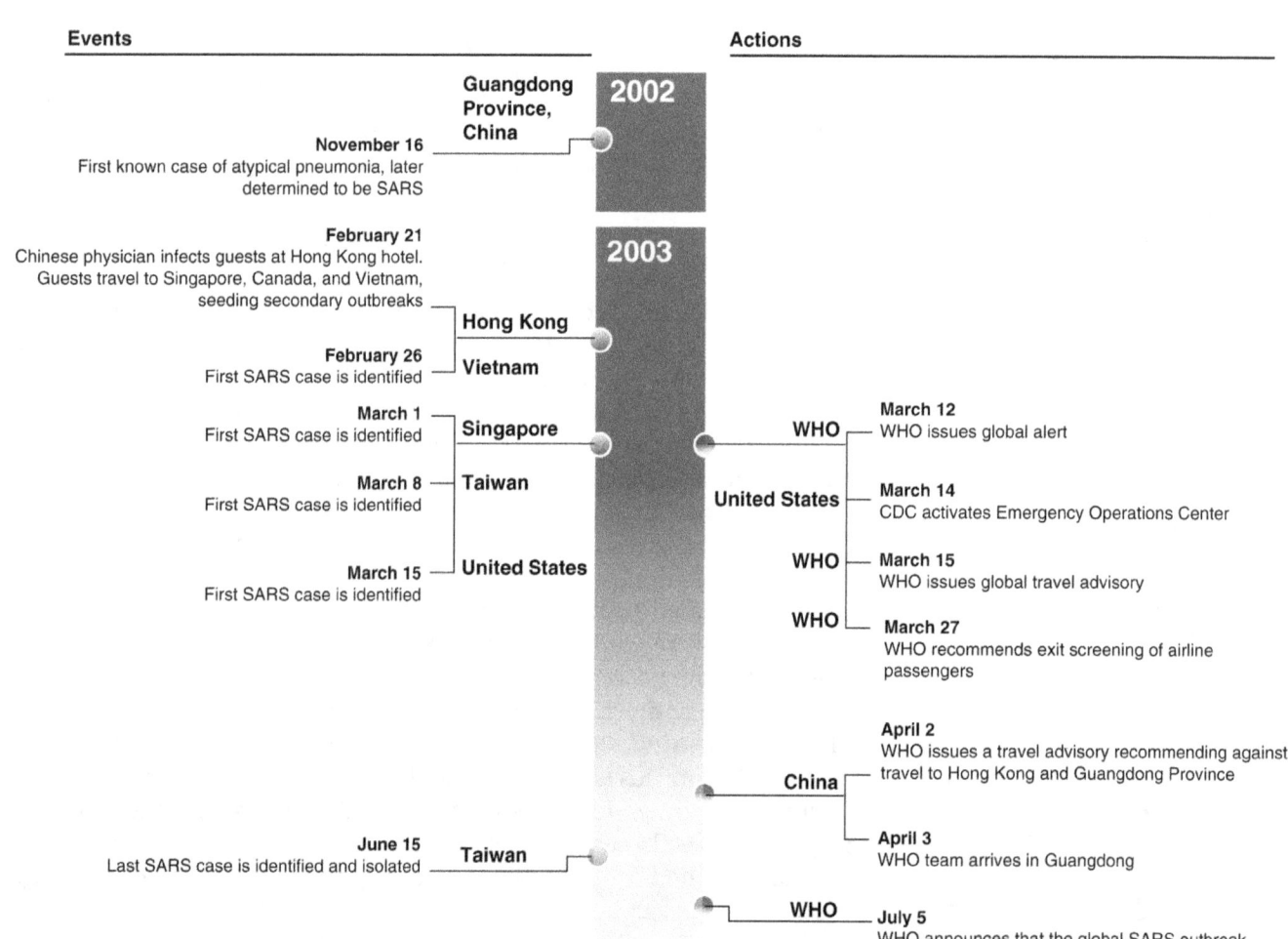

Events

November 16
First known case of atypical pneumonia, later determined to be SARS

Guangdong Province, China

2002

February 21
Chinese physician infects guests at Hong Kong hotel. Guests travel to Singapore, Canada, and Vietnam, seeding secondary outbreaks

2003

Hong Kong

February 26
First SARS case is identified

Vietnam

March 1
First SARS case is identified

Singapore

March 8
First SARS case is identified

Taiwan

March 15
First SARS case is identified

United States

June 15
Last SARS case is identified and isolated

Taiwan

Actions

WHO — **March 12**
WHO issues global alert

United States — **March 14**
CDC activates Emergency Operations Center

WHO — **March 15**
WHO issues global travel advisory

WHO — **March 27**
WHO recommends exit screening of airline passengers

April 2
WHO issues a travel advisory recommending against travel to Hong Kong and Guangdong Province

China

April 3
WHO team arrives in Guangdong

WHO — **July 5**
WHO announces that the global SARS outbreak has been contained

Source: GAO analysis of WHO data.

Global Infectious Disease Control and the Role of the World Health Organization

Although national governments bear primary responsibility for disease surveillance and response, WHO, an agency of the United Nations, plays a central role in global infectious disease control. WHO provides support, information, and recommendations to governments and the international community during outbreaks of infectious disease that threaten global health or trade. The International Health Regulations outline WHO's authority and member states' obligations in preventing the global spread of infectious diseases. Adopted in 1951 and last modified in 1981, the International Health Regulations are designed to ensure maximum security against the international spread of diseases with a minimum of interference with world traffic (that is, trade and travel). The current regulations require that member states report the incidence of three diseases within their borders—cholera, plague, and yellow fever—and WHO can investigate an outbreak only after receiving the consent of the government involved. Efforts to revise the regulations began in 1995, and the revised regulations are scheduled to be ready for submission to the World Health Assembly, the governing body of WHO, in May 2005.[4]

While the International Health Regulations provide the legal framework for global infectious disease control, WHO's Global Outbreak Alert and Response Network (GOARN), established in April 2000, is the primary mechanism by which WHO mobilizes technical resources for the investigation of, and response to, disease outbreaks of international importance. Because WHO does not have the human and financial resources to respond to all disease outbreaks, GOARN relies on the resources of its partners, including scientific and public health institutions in member states, surveillance and laboratory networks (e.g., WHO's Global Influenza Surveillance Network)[5], other U.N. organizations, the International Committee of the Red Cross, and international humanitarian nongovernmental organizations. WHO collects intelligence about outbreaks through various sources, including formal reports from governments and WHO officials in the field as well as informal reports from

---

[4]WHO, which consists of 192 member states, is headquartered in Geneva and has six regional offices and numerous country offices. The Western Pacific Regional Office (WPRO) serves Asian countries and has links to country offices in China and other Asian countries. WHO is governed by the World Health Assembly, which meets yearly and is attended by delegations from all member states. The assembly determines WHO's policies and is authorized to adopt regulations concerning the prevention of the international spread of disease and make recommendations about any subject dealt with by WHO. China is member of WHO, but Taiwan is not. Hong Kong's interests are represented in WHO by China.

[5]The influenza surveillance network comprises four WHO Collaborating Centers and 112 institutions in 83 countries, which are recognized by WHO as "WHO National Influenza Centers." The National Influenza Centers collect specimens in their country and perform primary virus isolation and characterization. They ship newly isolated strains to the Collaborating Centers for analysis, the result of which forms the basis for WHO recommendations on the composition of influenza vaccine for the Northern and Southern Hemisphere each year.

the media and the Internet.[6] When WHO receives a formal request for assistance from a national government, it responds primarily through GOARN. GOARN's key response objectives are to ensure that appropriate technical assistance rapidly reaches affected areas during an outbreak and to strengthen public health response capacity within countries for future outbreaks. Its response activities may include providing technical advice or support (e.g., public health experts and laboratory services), logistical aid (e.g., supplies and vaccines), and financial assistance (e.g., emergency funds). In addition to the support provided through GOARN, technical assistance and deployments are also arranged through WHO's regional offices.

U.S. Government Agencies Responsible for Responding to Global Infectious Disease Outbreaks

Two departments of the U.S. government, the Department of Health and Human Services (HHS) and State, play major roles in responding to infectious disease outbreaks overseas.[7] Within HHS, the Office of Global Health Affairs and CDC work closely with WHO and foreign governments in response efforts.[8] CDC also works with other federal agencies, state and local health departments, and the travel industry to limit the introduction of communicable diseases into the United States. State's roles include protecting U.S. government employees working overseas and disseminating information about situations that may pose a threat to U.S. citizens living and traveling abroad. In addition, State may coordinate the provision of technical assistance by various U.S. government agencies and use its diplomatic contacts to engage foreign governments on policy issues related to infectious disease response.

---

[6]About 40 percent of the approximately 200 outbreaks investigated and reported to WHO each year come from the Global Public Health Intelligence Network (GPHIN), a system developed by Canadian health officials and used by WHO since 1997 that searches for reports of disease outbreaks from more than 950 news feeds and discussion groups around the world in the media and on the Internet.

[7]The Departments of Defense, Homeland Security, and Transportation also assisted State and HHS during the SARS outbreak.

[8]The National Institute of Allergy and Infectious Diseases and the Food and Drug Administration also played roles in the response to SARS by conducting and supporting scientific research (e.g., on diagnostic tests and a vaccine) during and after the outbreak.

Infectious Disease Control in China, Hong Kong, and Taiwan

In recent years, Asia has become increasingly vulnerable to emerging infectious disease outbreaks, and governments have had to deal with diseases such as avian influenza and dengue fever. In China, Hong Kong, and Taiwan, such infectious disease outbreaks are managed through the public health authorities of these governments:

- *China:* The Ministry of Health maintains lead authority over health policy at the national level, although provincial governments exercise significant authority over local health matters. In January 2002, the national Center for Disease Control and Prevention was established, along with centers at the provincial and local levels, and charged with matters ranging from infectious disease control to chronic disease management.

- *Hong Kong:* The Health, Welfare, and Food Bureau has overall policy responsibility for health care delivery and other human services in Hong Kong. Within the bureau, the Department of Health and its Disease Prevention and Control Division, which was established in July 2000, are responsible for formulating strategies and implementing measures in the surveillance, prevention, and control of communicable diseases. The Hospital Authority is responsible for the management of 43 public hospitals in Hong Kong.

- *Taiwan:* The Department of Health is responsible for national health matters and for guiding, supervising, and coordinating local health bureaus. A division of the department, the Taiwan Center for Disease Control, was established in 1999 and consolidated the disease prevention work of several national public health agencies involved in infectious disease control.

WHO's Response to SARS Was Extensive, but Was Delayed by an Initial Lack of Cooperation from China and Challenged by Limited Resources

WHO's actions to respond to the SARS outbreak were extensive, but its response was delayed by an initial lack of cooperation from officials in China and challenged by limited resources. WHO's actions included direct technical assistance to affected areas and broad international actions such as alerting the international community about this serious disease and issuing information, guidance, and recommendations to government officials, health professionals, the general public, and the media. (See fig. 1 for key WHO actions during the SARS outbreak.) However, an initial lack of cooperation on the part of China limited WHO's access to information about the outbreak, and WHO had to stretch its resources for infectious disease control to capacity.

WHO Provided Direct Assistance to Affected Areas

WHO's response to SARS was coordinated jointly by WHO headquarters and its Western Pacific Regional Office (WPRO). At headquarters, WHO activated its GOARN. Although GOARN had been used before to respond to isolated outbreaks of Ebola, meningitis, viral hemorrhagic fever, and cholera in African countries and elsewhere, the SARS outbreak was the first time the network was activated on such a large scale for an international outbreak of an unknown emerging infectious disease. There were two primary aspects to WHO's activities during the SARS outbreak: One was the direct deployment of public health specialists from around the world to affected Asian governments to provide technical assistance; the other was the formation of three virtual networks of laboratory specialists, clinicians, and epidemiologists who pooled their knowledge, expertise, and resources to collect and develop the information WHO needed to issue its guidance and communications about SARS.

Deployment

Under GOARN's auspices, WHO rapidly deployed 115 specialists from 26 institutions in 17 countries to provide direct technical assistance to SARS-affected areas. WPRO also facilitated the deployment of an additional 80 public health specialists to SARS-affected areas. Asian governments identified their needs for technical assistance—consisting primarily of more senior, experienced staff—and then WHO issued a request for staff from its partners. WHO officials at headquarters and at WPRO worked jointly to quickly process contracts and send teams into the field within 48 hours of the request. The work of the teams varied, depending on local need. For example, a team of 5 public health experts sent to China reviewed clinical and epidemiologic data to improve the detection and surveillance of SARS cases in Guangdong. A team of 4 public health experts sent to Hong Kong included environmental engineers to help investigate the spread of SARS in a housing complex.

Virtual Networks

WHO also formed several international networks of researchers and clinicians, including a laboratory network, a clinical network, and an epidemiologic network. These networks operated "virtually," communicating through a secure Web site and teleconferences. The SARS laboratory network, based on the model of WHO's global influenza surveillance network and using some of the same laboratories, consisted of 13 laboratories in 9 countries. Within one month of its creation, participants in this network had identified the SARS coronavirus and shortly afterward sequenced its genome. The SARS clinical network consisted of more than 50 clinicians in 14 countries. Clinicians in this network helped to develop the SARS case definition and wrote infection control guidelines. The SARS epidemiologic network, which consisted of 32 epidemiologists from 11 institutions, collected data and conducted studies on the characteristics of SARS, including its transmission and control. WHO and other public health experts noted that there was a high level of collaboration and cooperation in these scientific networks.

WHO Alerted the International Community and Made Important Recommendations amid Scientific Uncertainty

During the SARS outbreak, WHO played a key role in alerting the world about the disease and issuing information, guidance, and recommendations to government officials, health professionals, the general public, and the media that helped raise awareness and control the outbreak.

Global Alerts and Travel Recommendations

When WHO became concerned about outbreaks of atypical pneumonia in China, Hong Kong, and Vietnam, it issued a global alert on March 12, 2003, warning the world about the appearance of a severe respiratory illness of undetermined cause that was rapidly spreading among health care workers. Three days later, on March 15, WHO issued a second, higher-level global alert in which it identified the disease as SARS and first published a definition of suspect and probable cases.[9] At the same time, WHO also issued its first emergency travel advisory to international travelers, calling on all travelers to be aware of the main symptoms of SARS. When, on March 27, it became clear to WHO that 27 cases of SARS were linked to exposure on five airline flights, WHO recommended the screening of air passengers on flights departing from areas where there was local transmission of SARS. On April 2, WHO began issuing travel advisories—

---

[9]At this time, WHO defined a suspect case as one occurring after February 1, 2003, with a history of a high fever (over 38 degrees Celsius) and one or more respiratory symptoms, including cough, shortness of breath, and difficulty breathing. It defined a probable case as one in which there was close contact with a person diagnosed with SARS; a history of recent travel to areas reporting SARS; a diagnosis of "suspect" with chest X-ray findings of pneumonia or respiratory distress syndrome; or an unexplained respiratory illness resulting in death, plus an autopsy examination demonstrating the pathology of respiratory distress syndrome without an identifiable cause. WHO revised this definition several times, publishing the latest revision on August 14, 2003 (see http://www.who.int/csr/sars/postoutbreak/en/).

recommendations that travelers should consider postponing all but essential travel to designated areas where the risk of exposure to SARS was considered high. The first designated areas were Hong Kong and Guangdong Province, China; later, the list was expanded to include other parts of China; Toronto; and Taiwan. During the SARS outbreak, WHO also publicized a list of areas with recent local transmission of SARS.

Guidelines and Recommendations on the Management of SARS

In addition to travel recommendations, WHO developed more than 20 other guidelines and recommendations for responding to SARS during the outbreak. These included advice on the detection and management of cases, laboratory diagnosis of SARS, hospital infection control, and how to handle mass gatherings of persons arriving from an area of recent local transmission of SARS. These guidelines and recommendations were disseminated through WHO's SARS Web site, which was updated regularly and received 6 million to 10 million hits per day.

WHO Faced Challenges in Issuing Guidance and Recommendations

In issuing guidance and recommendations about SARS, WHO had to respond immediately while making the best use of limited scientific knowledge about the disease (e.g., its cause, mode of transmission, and treatment), and it had to communicate effectively to public health professionals and the general public. This situation posed challenges, and WHO's efforts came under some criticism. For example, officials in Canada, Taiwan, and Hong Kong—areas that were directly affected by the travel recommendations—criticized WHO for not being more transparent in the process it used to issue and lift the recommendations. They also stated that the evidentiary foundation for issuing the recommendations was weak and the process did not allow countries enough time to prepare (e.g., to develop press releases and inform the tourism industry). WHO officials and others also acknowledged that communicating effectively about the risks of transmitting SARS and recommending appropriate action were major challenges for the organization. For example, even though WHO officials believed that the use of face masks by the general public was ineffective in preventing SARS, it had a difficult time communicating this fact and educating the general public about appropriate preventive measures. In addition, WHO recommended screening of airline passengers before departure, but the recommendation was vague and allowed countries to execute it in different ways.

Initial Lack of Cooperation from China Limited WHO's Access to Information and Delayed Its Response

Although WHO officials at headquarters and in the field received various informal reports of a serious outbreak of atypical pneumonia in China's Guangdong Province early in the SARS outbreak, WHO did not issue its global alerts until mid-March 2003. This delay occurred both because there was scientific uncertainty about the disease and because of initial lack of cooperation by China, which limited WHO's access to information and its ability to assist in investigating and managing the outbreak. As detailed in appendix II, WHO first received informal reports about a serious disease outbreak in Guangdong Province in November 2002. At the time, influenza was suspected as the primary cause of this outbreak. When WHO requested further information from Chinese authorities, it was told that influenza activity in China was normal and that there were no unusual strains of the virus. Despite WHO's repeated requests, Chinese authorities did not grant it permission to go to Guangdong Province and investigate the outbreak until April 2, 2003.

WHO lacked authority under the International Health Regulations to compel China to report the SARS outbreak and to allow WHO to assist in investigating and managing it. WHO officials told us that, in general, the organization tries to play a neutral, coordinating role and relies on government cooperation to investigate problems and ensure that appropriate control measures are being implemented. Vietnam, for example, cooperated with WHO early in the outbreak, which may have contributed to a less severe outbreak in that country. In the case of China, WHO exerted some pressure, as did the U.S. government, and the international media, which eventually helped persuade China to become more open about the situation and to allow WHO to assist in investigating and managing the outbreak.

WHO's Response to SARS Was Challenged by Limited Resources

While extensive, WHO's response to SARS in Asia was challenged by limited resources devoted to infectious disease control and in particular to GOARN. WHO's ability to respond in a timely and appropriate manner to outbreaks such as SARS is dependent upon the participation and support of WHO's partners and adequate financial support. During the SARS outbreak, GOARN's human resources were stretched to capacity. GOARN experienced difficulty in sustaining the response to SARS over time and getting the appropriate experts out into the field. WHO officials in China told us that they could not obtain experienced epidemiologists and hospital infection control experts and that ultimately they had to look outside the network to find assistance. GOARN was largely dependent on CDC staff to deploy to Asia to manage the epidemic response. According to a senior CDC official, if the United States had experienced many SARS cases during the global outbreak, CDC might not have been able to make as many of these staff available. Furthermore, some GOARN partners told us that the staffing requests that they received from GOARN, WPRO, and WHO country offices were not well coordinated. This issue was raised at a GOARN Steering Committee meeting in June 2003, and it was suggested that a stronger regional capacity for coordination could help ensure the necessary public health experts are mobilized and deployed to the field.

The SARS outbreak also highlighted the limitations in GOARN's financial resources. Historically, the network has received limited financial support from WHO's core budget, which consists of assessed contributions from members. The network tries to make up for shortfalls by soliciting additional contributions from member states, foundations, and other donors. There are limited resources to pay for headquarters staff and technical resources such as computer mapping software and to support management initiatives such as strategic planning and evaluation activities. While acknowledging that planning and evaluation are important both for responding to future outbreaks and for ensuring epidemic preparedness and capacity building, WHO officials told us that GOARN is usually focused on the response to an immediate emergency and thus lacks the time and resources to retrospectively review what worked well and what did not.

U.S. Government Had Key Role in Response to SARS, but Efforts Revealed Problems in Ability to Respond to Emerging Infectious Diseases

CDC, as part of HHS, and State played major roles in responding to the SARS outbreak, but their actions revealed limits in their ability to address emerging infectious diseases. CDC worked with WHO and Asian governments to identify and respond to the disease and helped limit its spread into the United States. However, CDC encountered obstacles that made it unable to trace international travelers because of airline concerns over CDC's authority and the privacy of passenger information, as well as procedural issues. State applied diplomatic pressure to governments, helped facilitate U.S. government efforts to respond to SARS in Asia, and supported U.S. government employees and citizens in the region. However, State encountered multiple difficulties in helping to arrange medical evacuations for U.S. citizens infected with SARS overseas. Based in part on this experience, State ultimately authorized departure of all nonessential U.S. government employees at several Asian posts.

CDC Played Central Role in Fighting SARS in Asia

Throughout the SARS outbreak, CDC was the foremost participant in WHO's multilateral efforts to recognize and respond to SARS in Asia, with CDC officials constituting about two-thirds of the 115 public health experts deployed to the region under the umbrella of GOARN. CDC also contributed its expertise and resources to epidemiological, laboratory, and clinical research on SARS. According to CDC, its involvement in recognizing the disease began in February 2003, when CDC officials joined WHO efforts to identify the cause of atypical pneumonia outbreaks in southern China, Vietnam, and Hong Kong. In March 2003, CDC set up an emergency operations center to coordinate sharing of information with WHO's epidemiology, clinical, and laboratory networks (see fig. 1). Under GOARN's auspices, CDC also assigned epidemiologists, laboratory scientists, hospital infection control specialists, and environmental engineers to provide technical assistance in Asia. For example, CDC assigned senior epidemiologists to help a WHO team investigate the outbreak in China. The team met with public health officials and health care workers in affected provinces to determine how they were responding to SARS. It also recommended steps to bring the outbreak under control, such as hospital infection control measures, quarantine strategies, and free health care for individuals with suspected SARS.

In addition, because Taiwan is not a member of WHO, CDC gave direct assistance to support Taiwan's response to SARS, serving as a link between Taiwanese health authorities and WHO and providing technical information and expertise that enabled Taiwan to control the outbreak. Shortly after Taiwan identified its first case of SARS imported from China in March 2003, Taiwanese authorities asked WHO for assistance. WHO officials transmitted the request to CDC and asked it to respond. Between March and July 2003, 30 CDC experts traveled to Taiwan and advised health authorities on various aspects of the SARS response. CDC epidemiologists recommended changes in Taiwan's approach to classifying SARS cases, which was time consuming and resulted in a large backlog of cases awaiting review as the outbreak expanded. They advised Taiwanese health authorities to replace their case classification system with a two-tiered approach that would categorize patients with SARS-like symptoms as either "suspect" or "probable" SARS. This strategy enabled public health authorities to institute precautionary control measures, such as isolation, for suspected SARS patients, and according to senior CDC and Taiwanese officials, it helped reduce transmission, including within medical facilities, and stop the outbreak.

CDC Took Actions to Limit Spread of SARS into the United States

When WHO issued its global SARS alert on March 12, 2003, CDC officials attempted to limit the disease's spread into the United States by (1) providing information for people traveling to or from SARS-affected areas and (2) ensuring that travelers arriving at U.S. borders with SARS-like symptoms received proper medical treatment. Beginning in mid-March 2003, CDC posted regular SARS updates on its Web site for people traveling to SARS-affected countries. At the same time, CDC's Division of Global Migration and Quarantine deployed quarantine officers to U.S. airports, seaports, and land crossings where travelers entered the United States from SARS-affected areas. The officers distributed health alert notices to all arriving travelers and crew (see fig. 2).

Figure 2: CDC Health Alert Notice

HEALTH ALERT NOTICE
Health Alert Notice for International Travelers
Arriving in the United States
from China, Vietnam, and Singapore

TO THE TRAVELER: During your recent travel, you may have been exposed to cases of severe acute respiratory disease syndrome (SARS). You should monitor your health for at least 10 days. If you become ill with fever, cough, or difficulty in breathing, you should consult a physician. In advance of your visit to the physician, tell him or her about your recent travel to these regions and whether you were in contact with someone who had these symptoms. Please save this card and give it to your physician if you become ill.

TO THE PHYSICIAN: The patient presenting this card may have recently traveled to China, Vietnam, or Singapore, where cases of SARS have been identified. If you suspect that this patient may have SARS, please contact your city, county, or state health officer (see http://www.cdc.gov or call the CDC Emergency Operations Center at 770-488-7100).

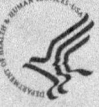 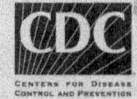

DEPARTMENT OF HEALTH AND HUMAN SERVICES

Source: Centers for Disease Control and Prevention.

The notices, printed in eight languages and describing SARS symptoms, incubation period, and what to do if symptoms developed, also contained a message to physicians to contact a public health officer or CDC if they treated a patient who might have SARS. CDC staff distributed close to 3 million health alert notices over a 3-month period. Department of Homeland Security staff assisted CDC by passing out the notices at land crossings between the United States and Canada. CDC's quarantine officers also responded to dozens of reports of passengers with SARS-like symptoms on airplanes and ships arriving in the United States from overseas. The officers boarded the airplane or ship, assessed the ill individuals to determine if they might have SARS and, if necessary, arranged the individuals' transport to a medical facility.

Regulatory, Privacy, and Procedural Concerns Hampered CDC's Efforts to Trace Travelers

CDC officials wanted to advise passengers who had traveled on an airplane or ship with a suspected SARS case to monitor themselves for SARS symptoms during the virus's 10-day incubation period, but due to airline concerns over authority and privacy, as well as procedural constraints, CDC was unable to obtain the passenger contact information it needed to trace travelers. Although HHS has statutory authority to prevent the introduction, transmission, or spread of communicable diseases from foreign countries into the United States,[10] HHS regulations implementing the statute do not specifically provide for HHS to obtain passenger manifests or other passenger contact information from airlines and shipping companies for disease outbreak control purposes.[11] CDC officials told us that some airlines failed to provide necessary contact information to CDC, which may be attributable to the lack of specific regulations in this area. Moreover, CDC officials said that in response to their requests, some airlines refused to give CDC passenger contact information from frequent flier databases or credit card receipts because of privacy concerns.[12] Even when CDC was able to obtain passenger information, CDC staff responsible for contacting travelers found passenger data untimely (because some airlines provided it after SARS's 10-day incubation period), insufficient (because some airlines could provide only passenger names but no contact information), or difficult to use (because it was available on paper rather than electronically). According to senior CDC officials, the inability to trace travelers who might have been exposed to SARS could have hampered their ability to limit the disease's spread into the United States.

---

[10]Section 361 of the Public Health Service Act, 42 U.S.C. § 264.

[11]See 42 C.F.R. pts 70 and 71; 21 C.F.R. pts 1240 and 1250.

[12]According to airline industry association officials, under European Union privacy laws and regulations, there could be problems with sharing passenger names and addresses with government agencies.

CDC Exploring Options to Resolve Tracing Problems

The obstacles to tracing travelers remain unresolved, and senior CDC officials are concerned they will encounter difficulties in limiting the spread of infectious diseases into the United States during future global infectious disease outbreaks.[13] CDC officials told us they are exploring several options to overcome the problems they encountered during the SARS outbreak. CDC may adopt one or more of these options,[14] including: clarifying CDC's authority by promulgating regulations specifically to obtain passenger contact information; coordinating with the Department of Homeland Security and other federal agencies for this purpose; developing a memorandum of understanding with airlines on sharing passenger information; and creating a system for obtaining passenger contact information in an electronic format. However, CDC officials said they have already faced obstacles in pursuing some of these options. For example, both CDC and Department of Homeland Security officials told us that Homeland Security's computer-based passenger information system could not be used for purposes other than national security.

State Applied Diplomatic Pressure, Helped Facilitate Agency Responses, and Disseminated Information

State also played an important role in the U.S. response to SARS, primarily by applying diplomatic pressure, helping facilitate government efforts overseas, and disseminating information. In March 2003, the U.S. Ambassador to China communicated with Chinese government officials to encourage China to be more transparent in reporting SARS cases and to grant WHO and CDC officials access to southern China. State also established two working groups to facilitate the U.S. government response to SARS in Asia. The first working group, comprising various State offices and bureaus, issued daily reports on the status of the outbreak to U.S. embassies and consulates. The second working group, established in May 2003, convened various U.S. government agencies, including State, HHS, and the Departments of Defense and Homeland Security, to address policy and response issues. U.S. government officials agreed that State's efforts helped provide valuable information during an uncertain period and

---

[13]During the SARS outbreak, international travelers constituted an important source of transmission. For example, CDC reported that all of the United States' eight laboratory-confirmed SARS cases and almost all of the 27 probable SARS cases were found in individuals who had traveled to a SARS-affected area or came into close contact with someone who did.

[14]CDC did not provide us with details about the various options because they had not yet been finalized.

allowed for a unified response to the outbreak. U.S. embassies and consulates in Asia also disseminated information to U.S. government employees and U.S. citizens living and traveling abroad. For example, they publicized CDC updates on SARS through e-mail alerts and on their Web sites and informed U.S. citizens about medical care available in-country.

State Faced Obstacles Arranging Medical Evacuations for U.S. Citizens with Suspected SARS

During the outbreak, even the strongest local health care systems were overwhelmed, and State was concerned that U.S. government employees might receive treatment that did not meet U.S. standards. For example, in Hong Kong and China, U.S. consular staff told us they were concerned about sending U.S. government employees to local hospitals because of inadequate infection control practices, limited availability of health care workers with English language skills, and controversial treatment protocols such as administering steroids to SARS patients.

In a few cases, State worked with private medical evacuation companies to help arrange medical evacuations for U.S. citizens with suspected SARS.[15] However, early in the outbreak, CDC had not yet developed guidelines to prevent transmission during flight, and medical evacuation companies could not obtain aircraft and crew willing to transport SARS patients because of the perceived health risks.[16] Even after CDC developed guidelines, medical evacuation companies still had difficulty finding aircraft because only about 5 percent of existing air ambulances could comply with the stringent guidelines, according to a private air medical evacuation official. Furthermore, a U.S. state and some medical facilities in the United States refused to accept SARS patients brought from Asia. For example, the state of Hawaii initially said it would accept medically evacuated SARS patients but later reneged and prevented one air ambulance company from bringing a U.S. citizen with suspected SARS to a

---

[15]State officials said they are responsible for providing medical services (including medical evacuations, if necessary) only to certain U.S. government employees and their dependents, although embassies may assist U.S. citizens overseas in obtaining medical care on a case-by-case basis. However, it is primarily the responsibility of U.S. citizens to arrange their own medical evacuation. During the SARS outbreak, State helped arrange three medical evacuations for U.S. citizens. The first was performed by the Department of Defense from Hanoi to Taiwan; the second was a land evacuation performed by ambulance from Shenzhen to Hong Kong; and the third was performed by a medical evacuation company from Taiwan to Atlanta.

[16]Most medical evacuation companies do not have their own aircraft and crews; rather, they subcontract aircraft as medical evacuation needs arise.

medical facility in Honolulu. Although the Department of Defense (Defense) performed one medical evacuation for a U.S. civilian under special circumstances, officials at State and Defense told us that military priorities and scarce resources are likely to prevent Defense from performing civilian evacuations in the future. Ultimately, State concluded that inadequate local health care and difficulties arranging medical evacuations put U.S. government employees at risk, and, in turn, State authorized departure for nonessential employees and their dependents at several posts.[17]

Medical Evacuation Issues Still Pose Challenges for Future Outbreaks

State has not developed a strategy to overcome the challenges that staff encountered in arranging international medical evacuations during the SARS outbreak, but it is working with other U.S. government agencies to develop guidance on this issue. Officials at State, CDC, Defense, and medical evacuation companies told us that the same obstacles could resurface during a new outbreak of SARS or another unknown infectious disease with airborne transmission. State officials said the medical evacuation companies that provide State's medical evacuation services have agreed to evacuate SARS patients, and the companies with whom we spoke confirmed that since the SARS outbreak, they have identified sufficient aircraft and crew to transport a limited number of patients. The exact number would depend on the nature of the disease, the patient's condition, and the type of medical care required. State officials said they have not investigated how many SARS patients private medical evacuation companies or Defense could transport; they also do not know which U.S. states and medical facilities would accept patients with SARS or another emerging infectious disease. State officials are concerned about a scenario in which dozens of staff at a U.S. embassy or consulate contract SARS or another infectious disease, in which case medical evacuation would probably not be feasible given the current constraints. This would also pose a problem if many U.S. citizens living or traveling overseas contracted such a disease. Private medical evacuation companies acknowledged that they might not be able to transport large numbers of patients; furthermore, they are unsure which destinations in the United States would accept patients with an infectious disease such as SARS. State officials said they are working with other U.S. government agencies to develop guidelines for consular staff to arrange international medical evacuations. However, it is

---

[17]When warranted by conditions at an overseas post, State can authorize U.S. government employees and their dependents to depart the post.

not clear that this guidance will resolve some of the obstacles encountered during the SARS outbreak. For example, a CDC official said the agency is working with medical facilities near international ports of entry to identify treatment destinations for medically evacuated patients with quarantinable infectious diseases such as SARS, but no agreements have been reached yet.

After Initial Struggle, Asian Governments Brought SARS Outbreak under Control

The Asian governments we studied initially struggled to respond to SARS but ultimately brought the outbreak under control. As acknowledged by Asian government officials, poor communication within China and between China and Hong Kong, Taiwan, and WHO obscured the severity of the outbreak during its initial stages. As the extent of the outbreak was recognized, the large-scale response to SARS in China, Hong Kong, and Taiwan was hindered by an initial lack of leadership and coordination. Further, weaknesses in disease surveillance systems, public health capacity, and hospital infection control limited the ability of Asian governments to track the number of cases of SARS and implement an effective response. Improved screening, rapid isolation of suspected cases, enhanced hospital infection control, and quarantine of close contacts ultimately helped end the outbreak. In the aftermath of SARS, efforts are under way to improve public health capacity in Asia to better deal with SARS and other infectious disease outbreaks.

Poor Communication Limited Information on Severity of SARS Outbreak in China

The Chinese government's poor communication within the country, with Hong Kong and Taiwan, and with WHO limited the flow of information about the severity of the SARS outbreak in its initial stages. For example, the Ministry of Health did not widely circulate a report concerning the spread of atypical pneumonia (later determined to be SARS) in Guangdong Province. The report was produced by health officials in Guangdong Province on January 23, 2003—more than 2 weeks before the Ministry of Health's first official public announcement on the outbreak.[18] The report warned all hospitals in the province about the disease and provided advice to control its spread. Officials in Hong Kong, which directly borders the province, were not aware of the report, and a senior official in Taiwan,

---

[18]The report was released during the Chinese New Year Holiday. According to one official, the report may not have received significant attention from health officials on leave during the holiday.

which maintains significant travel and commercial ties with Guangdong Province, said Taiwan did not receive the report or any official communication about the outbreak. In addition, WHO did not receive this information. Officials in Guangdong Province told us they could not share this information outside of China because this is the responsibility of the Ministry of Health. Further, according to Chinese regulations on state secrets, information on widespread epidemics is considered highly classified.[19]

Chinese scientists also did not effectively communicate their findings about the cause of SARS early in the outbreak because of government restrictions. For example, as reported in a scientific journal and later confirmed in our own fieldwork, Chinese military researchers successfully identified the coronavirus as a potential cause of SARS in early March 2003, several weeks before a network of WHO researchers proved it was the cause of SARS.[20] One Chinese scientist directly involved in the effort told us that these researchers were instructed to defer to scientists at the Chinese Center for Disease Control and Prevention, who announced erroneously that *Chlamydia pneumoniae*, a type of bacteria, was responsible for the atypical pneumonia outbreak. In addition, we were told that these researchers were not permitted to communicate their findings on the coronavirus directly to WHO officials because only the Ministry of Health could communicate directly with WHO.

Communication problems persisted as late as April 2003, 5 months after the first cases occurred. On April 3, the Minister of Health announced that the outbreak was under effective control and that only 12 cases of SARS had been reported in Beijing. However, a physician working at a military hospital in Beijing wrote a letter to an Asian news magazine claiming that there were significantly more SARS cases in military hospitals and that hospital officials were told not to disclose information about SARS to the public. On April 15, in response to rumors of underreporting, WHO officials leading an investigation into the outbreak were granted permission to visit military hospitals but stated that they were not authorized to report their

[19]See People's Republic of China, Ministry of Health, "Explanation on Regulations on State Secrets in Health Work and Their Specific Classification and Scope," March 1, 1991, published in *Chinese Law & Government* 66 (2003) (Fei-Ling Wang trans).

[20]Martin Enserink"SARS in China: China's Missed Chance," *Science*, vol. 301, no. 5,631 (2003).

findings. By April 20, the Ministry of Health announced the existence of 339 previously undisclosed cases of SARS in Beijing.

An Initial Lack of Effective Leadership and Coordination in SARS-Affected Areas in Asia Hindered Response

As acknowledged by government officials, a lack of effective leadership and coordination within the governments of China, Hong Kong, and Taiwan early in the outbreak hindered attempts to organize an effective response to SARS. In China, provincial and local authorities maintained significant responsibility and autonomy in conducting epidemiological investigations of SARS but failed to coordinate with one another and national authorities early in the outbreak. However, as SARS spread into Beijing, the highest political leaders of the Chinese Communist Party, citing an increased number of cases and the impact on travel and trade, advised officials to be more forthcoming about SARS cases. The Ministry of Health also acknowledged the ministry's failure to introduce a unified mechanism for collecting information about the outbreak and setting guidance and requirements across the country. Soon after those announcements, the Minister of Health and Mayor of Beijing were dismissed from their posts for downplaying the extent of the outbreak, and the public health response was brought under stronger central control. A vice premier of the central government assumed control of the Ministry of Health and convened ministerial level officers to take the lead in the nationwide SARS control effort.

In Hong Kong, an expert committee convened after the outbreak to investigate the government's response questioned the leadership and coordination of the public health system.[21] For example, the committee found that responsibility for managing infectious disease outbreaks was spread throughout different departments within the Health, Welfare, and Food Bureau, with no single authority designated as the central decision-making body during outbreaks. The committee also stated that poor coordination between the hospital and public health system further complicated the response. For example, the Hospital Authority responded to an outbreak within a hospital without informing the Department of Health, which learned of the outbreak through media reports. Further, the Hospital Authority and Department of Health used separate databases

---

[21]"SARS in Hong Kong: From Experience to Action," (Hong Kong: SARS Expert Committee, October 2, 2003), http://www.sars-expertcom.gov.hk/english/reports/reports/reports_fullrpt.html (downloaded Oct. 3, 2003).

during the initial stages of the outbreak and could not communicate information on new cases in real time.

In Taiwan, a report by WHO stated that the initial response to SARS was managed by senior political figures who sometimes did not heed the advice of technical experts. Furthermore, WHO noted that the failure to follow the advice of public health experts delayed the decision-making process and slowed the response to the outbreak in Taiwan. Taiwanese government officials noted that the leadership of the public health system was weak during the outbreak. In addition, the process they used to classify SARS cases was too slow to isolate suspected or probable cases. As the outbreak worsened and spread into hospitals throughout Taiwan, the Minister of Health and the director of the Taiwan Center for Disease Control resigned over criticisms about failing to control the spread of SARS.

Weaknesses in Disease Surveillance Systems and Public Health Capacity Further Constrained Efforts

As Asian governments monitored the spread of SARS, weaknesses in disease surveillance systems, public health capacity, and hospital infection control caused delays and gaps in disease reporting, which further constrained the response.

Disease Surveillance Systems

In China, health officials at the provincial level and WHO advisers working in the country noted that data gathering systems established in the epicenter of the outbreak in Guangdong Province were strong. However, Chinese officials also found that the effectiveness of a national disease surveillance system established in 1998 was limited. For example, disease prevention staff below the county level did not have access to computer terminals to report the number of SARS cases and had to relay disease reports to central authorities by fax or mail. In addition, the computer-based system did not permit the reporting of suspect cases that were not yet confirmed. Further, protocols for reporting were time consuming, since information was sent through multiple levels of the public health system. For example, during the outbreak, reports from doctors of suspect SARS cases could take up to 7 days to reach local public health authorities. In Beijing, an executive vice minister stated that the large number of undetected cases of SARS patients occurred because they could not collect information on SARS cases that were spread across 70 hospitals in the city. In Taiwan, duplicative reporting between municipal and federal levels led to unclear data on the total number of cases throughout the island. A WHO official reported that the surveillance data were entered into formats that were difficult to analyze and could not inform the public health response.

In Hong Kong, a quickly established atypical pneumonia surveillance system detected early cases of severe pneumonia admitted into hospitals. However, the expert committee reviewing the response noted that the limited access to data from private sector health care providers and a lack of comprehensive laboratory surveillance made it difficult for public health authorities to gain accurate information about the full extent of the outbreak and implement necessary control measures.

Public Health Capacity

In China, officials told us that a lack of funding and a reliance on market forces to finance public health services have weakened the country's ability to respond to outbreaks. For example, the newly established Center for Disease Control and Prevention system in China derives more than 50 percent of its revenue from user fees for immunizations and other services. WHO noted that the dependence on user fees has drawn attention and resources away from nonrevenue producing activities, such as disease surveillance, that are important for responding to infectious disease outbreaks. Furthermore, China did not have enough public health workers skilled in investigating diseases, and thus staff who had never been involved in disease investigations were used to trace SARS contacts and did not always collect the correct data on these cases. In Hong Kong, the expert committee noted that there was a shortage of expertise in field epidemiology and inadequate support for information systems. In addition, the committee found disproportionate funding of public health services compared with the public hospital system, which receives 10 times more government funds. Taiwanese officials cited problems in public health infrastructure, including the lack of equipment to deal with infectious patients in hospitals and underfunded laboratories.

Hospital Infection Control

Another major weakness in public health capacity cited by health officials in China, Hong Kong, and Taiwan was a lack expertise in hospital infection control. In many SARS-affected areas, transmission of SARS to health care workers and other hospital patients was a significant factor sustaining the outbreak. In some instances, hundreds of hospital-acquired infections were due to inadequate isolation of individual patients and limited availability and use of personal protective equipment (masks, gowns, and gloves) for hospital workers. For example, in Taiwan, health officials reported that after initial success in rapidly identifying and isolating cases arriving from other SARS-affected areas, hospitals failed to recognize SARS cases occurring within Taiwan, resulting in a secondary, and much larger, outbreak in hospitals throughout the island. WHO, U.S. CDC, and Taiwanese officials told us that the number of physicians trained in infection control practices was inadequate and that infection control was not a priority for hospital management. In Hong Kong, the expert committee noted that there was no clear leadership from infection control doctors and that there were insufficient numbers of nurses trained in hospital infection control.[22] In China, WHO officials noted in field reports that infection control procedures were rudimentary and relied on a range of measures, including disinfection of health care facilities, instead of the recommended isolation measures needed to limit spread to patients and health care workers.

Basic Public Health Strategies Eventually Worked to Control SARS Outbreak

The SARS outbreak was ultimately brought under control by a more coordinated response that included the implementation of basic public health strategies. Measures such as improved screening and reporting of cases, rapid isolation of SARS patients, enhanced hospital infection control practices, and quarantine of close contacts were the most effective ways to break the chain of person-to-person transmission.

Improved Screening and Reporting

Screening of patients with symptoms of SARS permitted the early identification of suspect cases during the early phase of illness. Furthermore, because SARS is transmitted when individuals have symptoms of the disease, detecting symptomatic patients was considered critical to stopping its spread. For example, in Beijing, fever clinics were established to screen people with fevers before presentation to hospitals or other health care providers to limit exposure to SARS. Between May 7 and June 9, 2003, there were 65,321 fever clinic visits. Through this effort, 47 probable SARS cases were identified, representing only 0.1 percent of all fever clinic visits but 84 percent of all probable cases hospitalized during that period. In addition, policies were implemented requiring daily reports from all areas regardless of whether any SARS cases were found. In Hong Kong, designated medical centers were established to conduct medical monitoring of close contacts of SARS patients to ensure early detection of secondary cases. In Taiwan, hospital staff and other individuals who had contact with SARS patients in hospitals were monitored on a daily basis to detect SARS symptoms.

Rapid Isolation and Contact Tracing

The identification of patients with suspect and probable cases of SARS and their close contacts reduced the rate of contact between SARS patients and

---

[22]SARS Expert Committee Report, "SARS in Hong Kong: From Experience to Action."

healthy individuals in both community and hospital settings. For example, toward the end of the outbreak, one Chinese province decreased the average time between onset of SARS symptoms to hospitalization from 4 days to 1, and the time to trace contacts of these patients from 1 day to less than half a day. These declines in the time for hospitalization and contact tracing generally coincided with a decrease in the number of new cases. In Hong Kong, officials facilitated tracing by linking a SARS database used by public health officials with police databases to track and verify the addresses of relatives and other close contacts of SARS patients. To limit the spread of SARS in the hospital system, specific hospitals were designated to treat suspected SARS patients in all SARS-affected areas. Another strategy in SARS-affected areas was the cancellation of school, large public gatherings, and holiday activities. For example, in China the weeklong May Day celebration was shortened.

Enhanced Hospital Infection Control

The widespread use of personal protective equipment helped contain the spread of SARS in hospitals. For example, in China, when hospital infection control measures were instituted toward the end of the outbreak in a 1,000-bed hospital constructed exclusively for SARS patients, there were no further cases of SARS transmission in health care workers. Similarly in Hong Kong and Taiwan, these measures led to a decline in the number of infections in health care workers. In addition, in all these affected areas, guidelines were ultimately established for the use of personal protective equipment in outbreak situations.

Quarantine Measures

China, Taiwan, and Hong Kong implemented quarantine measures to isolate potentially infected individuals from the larger community, which, when restricted to close contacts of SARS patients, proved to be an efficient and effective public health strategy. In Hong Kong, for example, close contacts of SARS patients and people in high-risk areas were isolated for 10 days in designated medical centers or at home to ensure early detection of secondary cases. However, more wide-scale quarantine took place in Taiwan, where 131,000 individuals who had any form of contact with a SARS patient or traveled to SARS-affected areas were placed under quarantine, and in Beijing, where more than 30,000 people were quarantined. Analysis of data from these areas indicated that the quarantine of individuals with no close contact to SARS patients was not an effective use of resources. For example, among the 133 probable and suspect cases identified in Taiwan, most were found to have had direct contact with a SARS patient.[23] Similarly, researchers found that in Beijing, limiting quarantine to close contacts of actively ill patients would have been a more efficient strategy and a better use of resources.[24]

Asian Governments Have Efforts Under Way to Build Public Health Capacity for Future Outbreaks

Following the SARS epidemic, Asian governments have attempted to improve public health capacity, revise their legal frameworks for infectious disease control, increase regional communication and cooperation, and utilize international aid to improve preparedness. During our fieldwork, we met with public health representatives at various levels—from senior health ministry officials to local hospital health care workers—who provided information on efforts to improve public health capacity. For example, after the SARS outbreak the Chinese government provided additional budgetary support and expanded authority to improve coordination and communication. The government also devised a plan to build capacity in its weak rural health care system. In Hong Kong, the government focused its efforts on early detection and response to infectious disease outbreaks and is developing a Center for Health Protection focused on infectious disease control. Several drills were conducted to test the system, and the government has identified protecting populations in senior citizen homes, schools, and hospitals as a priority. In Taiwan, the government responded to public health management shortcomings by establishing a new public health command structure with centralized authority and decision-making power and making numerous changes in health leadership positions. The government invested public funds to upgrade its health infrastructure—for example, to construct fever wards, isolation rooms with negative pressure relative to the surrounding area, and other improvements in hospitals.

The SARS outbreak also led to legal reforms specific to SARS control and the function of public health systems in SARS-affected areas. For example, China, Hong Kong, and Taiwan passed legislation or regulations during the outbreak that required clinicians and public health authorities to report cases of SARS. In China, regulations on the prevention of SARS were passed that, among other things, were intended to improve communication

---

[23]"Use of Quarantine to Prevent Transmission of Severe Acute Respiratory Syndrome—Taiwan 2003," *MMWR*, vol. 52, no. 29 (July 25, 2003).

[24]"Efficiency of Quarantine during an Epidemic of Severe Acute Respiratory Syndrome—Beijing, China 2003," *MMWR*, vol. 52, no. 43 (Oct. 31, 2003).

with the public and outline administrative or criminal penalties for officials who do not report SARS cases. [25] A broader set of regulations that may have a long-term impact was also passed that requires the creation of a unified command during public health emergencies, reporting of such emergencies within 2 hours, and improved public health capacity at all levels of the government.[26] In Hong Kong, the law was revised to enhance the power of public health authorities to isolate cases and control the spread of SARS through international travel.[27]

Senior government officials have taken steps to improve public health communication and coordination in the region. Health officials in Hong Kong and Taiwan stated it is critical that information on disease outbreaks in mainland China be quickly reported so that neighboring governments can take preventive actions. A post-SARS agreement among Guangdong Province, Hong Kong, and Macau has thus far led to monthly sharing of information on a list of 30 diseases. A senior Chinese health official stated that the SARS outbreak taught the Chinese government the need for international cooperation in fighting infectious disease outbreaks. According to WHO officials, since the 2002-2003 SARS outbreak, they have experienced increased transparency and willingness on the part of the Chinese government to work with WHO health experts.

The international community and the United States have committed financial and human resources to support the recent financial investments in public health capacity made by the Chinese government. For example, in July 2003 the World Bank announced a multidonor-supported program to strengthen disease surveillance and reporting and improve the skills of clinicians in China. The program is funded by US$11.5 million in loans from the World Bank, a 3 million British pound grant from the United Kingdom's Department for International Development, a Can$5 million grant from the Canadian International Development Agency, and a US$2 million regional grant from the Japan Social Development Fund. HHS is in the process of

---

[25]People's Republic of China, "Regulations for the Management of Infectious Atypical Pneumonia," May 13, 2003, published in 36 *Chinese Law & Government* 91(2003) (Fei-Ling Wang, trans).

[26]People's Republic of China, "Regulations on Contingency Measures for Public Health Emergencies," May 9, 2003, published in 36 *Chinese Law and Government* 76 (2003) (Fei-Ling Wang,tran).

[27]Laws of Hong Kong, Prevention of the Spread of Infectious Diseases, ch. 141B, regs. 27A and 27B (Apr. 17, 2003).

finalizing a multiyear, multimillion-dollar program of cooperation between HHS and the Chinese Ministry of Health aimed at strengthening China's capacity in public health management, epidemiology, and laboratory capacity. As part of the initiative, CDC staff members will be stationed in China to help strengthen the epidemiology workforce.

SARS Outbreak Decreased Consumer Confidence and Negatively Affected a Number of Asian Economies

During the SARS outbreak, consumer confidence temporarily declined as a result of consumer fears about SARS and precautions taken to avoid contracting the disease. This decline in consumer confidence in turn led to economic losses in Asian economies estimated in the billions of dollars. Service sectors were hit the hardest due to declines in travel and tourism to areas with SARS outbreaks and declines in retail sales involving face-to-face exchanges. Additionally, to counter economic losses associated with SARS, many Asian governments implemented costly economic stimulus programs.

Impacts from SARS Are Estimated to Have Cost Billions, Although Most Economies Have Recovered

While the number of cases and associated medical costs for the SARS outbreak were relatively low compared with those for other major historical epidemics, the economic costs of SARS were significant because they derived primarily from fears about the disease and precautions to avoid the disease, rather than the disease itself. As shown in table 1, one industry and one official estimate of the economic cost of SARS in Asia calculated the net loss in total output at roughly $11 billion to $18 billion, respectively. (These estimates reflect changes in growth forecasts that were calculated concurrent with the outbreak. See app. III for a discussion of methodologies and varied assumptions used to obtain these estimates.) For example, the *Far Eastern Economic Review* estimates SARS's economic costs in Asia at around $11 billion, with the largest losses in China, Hong Kong, and Singapore. The Asian Development Bank also shows the largest losses in these three economies, although they estimate the total cost at around $18 billion.[28] As the Asian Development Bank reported, using its cost estimate, the cost per person infected with SARS was roughly $2 million. While economic costs associated with a general loss in consumer confidence are difficult to quantify exactly, they illustrate

---

[28]These figures represent the net loss in GDP and take into account the potential decline in imports that acts to partially offset the potential decline in consumption or exports. As such, if the total loss in spending, rather than the net loss in GDP, is estimated, the Asian Development Bank's cost estimate rises to $60 billion.

how emerging diseases and fears associated with those diseases can have widespread ramifications for a large number of economies.

Table 1: Estimated Economic Cost of SARS in Asia

U.S. dollars in millions

	Far Eastern Economic Review	Asian Development Bank
China	2,200	6,100
Hong Kong	1,700	4,600
Malaysia	660	400
Singapore	950	2,700
Taiwan	820	1,300
Thailand	490	1,900
Vietnam	111	400
Region	10,700	18,000

Source: GAO analysis of data from *Far Eastern Economic Review* and Asian Development Bank.

Note: Regional totals may include costs in Asian countries other than those listed in the table.

The economic cost of SARS in terms of a percentage loss in each selected Asian economy's GDP has also been estimated by the Asian Development Bank and industry organizations at roughly 0.5 percent to 2 percent, with some variation among economies depending upon the importance of affected sectors in total output (see app. III for a more detailed discussion of these models' assumptions and their GDP loss estimates per country).[29] Figure 3 shows quarterly GDP growth for four Asian economies most affected by SARS—China, Hong Kong, Singapore, and Taiwan—and illustrates that GDP weakened in the second quarter of 2003, concurrent with the height of the SARS outbreak.[30] However, given that the outbreak was brought under control by July 2003, the economic impacts were

---

[29]Some economies were more vulnerable to SARS than others due to structural issues, such as the relative share of tourism in the economy, government spending responses, and prior consumer sentiment. For example, Hong Kong and Singapore have larger estimated GDP losses due to SARS because of weakened consumption demand already apparent in late 2002.

[30]We cannot, however, attribute viewed changes in quarterly GDP growth exclusively to SARS, given that other factors were relevant, such as the conflict in Iraq. Nonetheless, comparing Asian GDP growth rates with the average growth rate in Organization for Economic Cooperation and Development countries shows a much more distinct decline in the second quarter of 2003.

concentrated primarily in this second quarter. In fact, when WHO declared that the SARS outbreak was over in July 2003, pent-up demand during the outbreak likely contributed to an economic rebound in the third and fourth quarters.

Figure 3: Quarterly GDP Growth for Various Asian Economies, 2002-2003

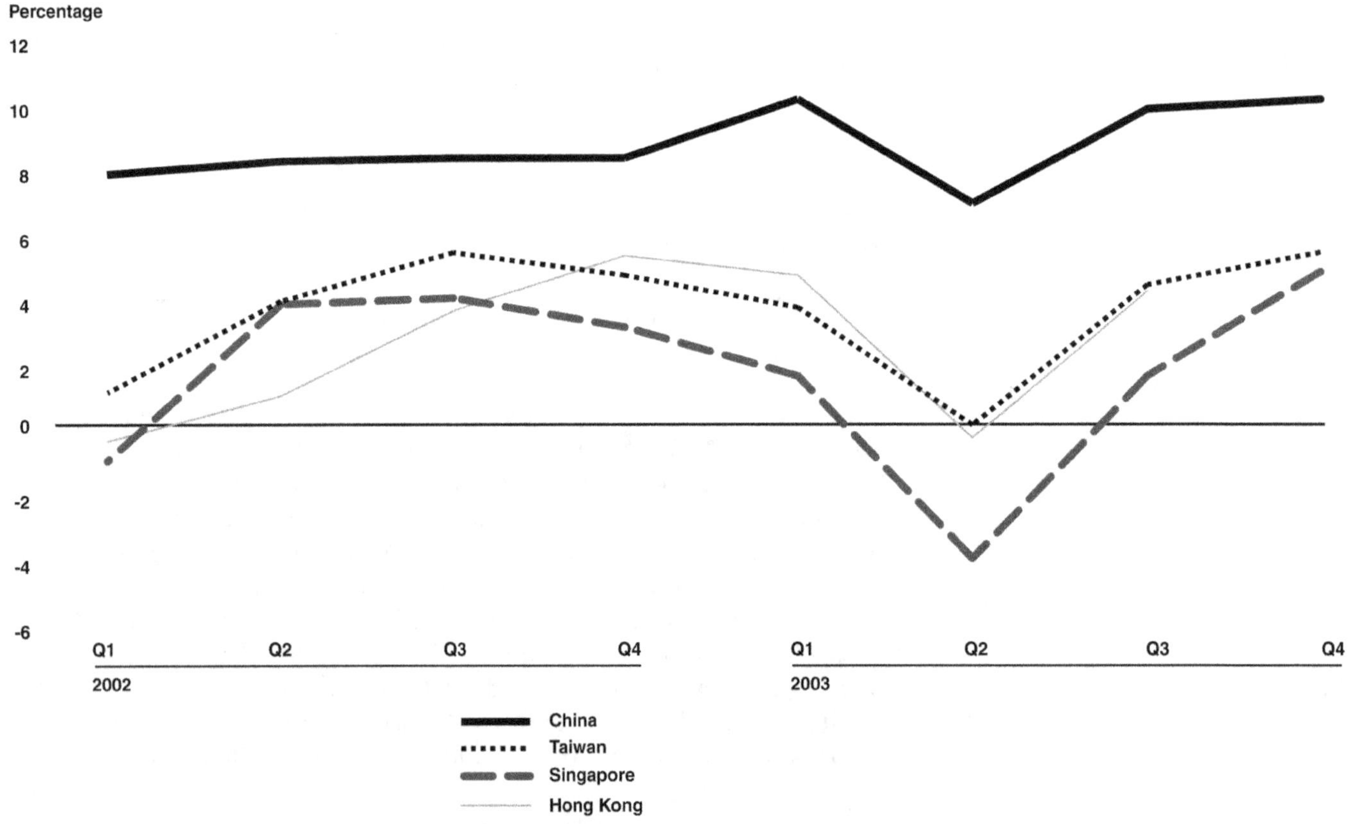

Percentage

Source: GAO analysis of data from national statistical offices in China, Hong Kong, Singapore, and Taiwan.

SARS Affected Asian Economies through a Variety of Channels

The SARS outbreak produced negative impacts on Asian economies through a variety of mechanisms. The most important channel through which SARS affected these economies was by temporarily dampening consumer confidence, particularly in the travel and tourism industry. In addition, decreased consumer confidence likely reduced retail sales and, to a lesser extent, some foreign trade and investment. Due to reduced demand, employment in affected economies fell. Some businesses also reported an increase in costs as business operations were disrupted, international shipments of goods and trade were hampered, and disease prevention costs rose.

The most severe economic impacts from SARS occurred in the travel and tourism industry, with airlines being particularly hard hit. As shown in figure 4, declines in regional airline traffic reached 40 percent to 50 percent in April and May, two months in which WHO travel advisories for Asia Pacific were in effect.[31] The estimated percentage decline in overall tourism earnings amounted to 15 percent in Vietnam, 25 percent in China, and more than 40 percent in Hong Kong and Singapore, according to the World Travel and Tourism Council.[32] Estimated job losses resulting from these SARS-related impacts were also significant. For example, the World Travel and Tourism Council estimated tourism sector job losses of around 27,000 in Hong Kong and 18,000 in Singapore, while the World Bank estimated airline job losses in the region at around 36,000.[33]

---

[31]As with the quarterly decline in GDP, we cannot attribute the entire decrease in airline traffic to SARS, as the outbreak occurred during an already depressed market because of the war in Iraq.

[32]The World Travel and Tourism Association used its own model to generate its estimates for the dollars lost from the decline in tourism. As such, these numbers do not correspond equally to the estimates in table 1.

[33]The duration of estimated job losses is unknown. Travel and tourism in Asia has largely recovered, and International Airline Traffic Association forecasts for the industry are optimistic.

Figure 4: Estimated Economic Impacts of SARS on Travel and Tourism

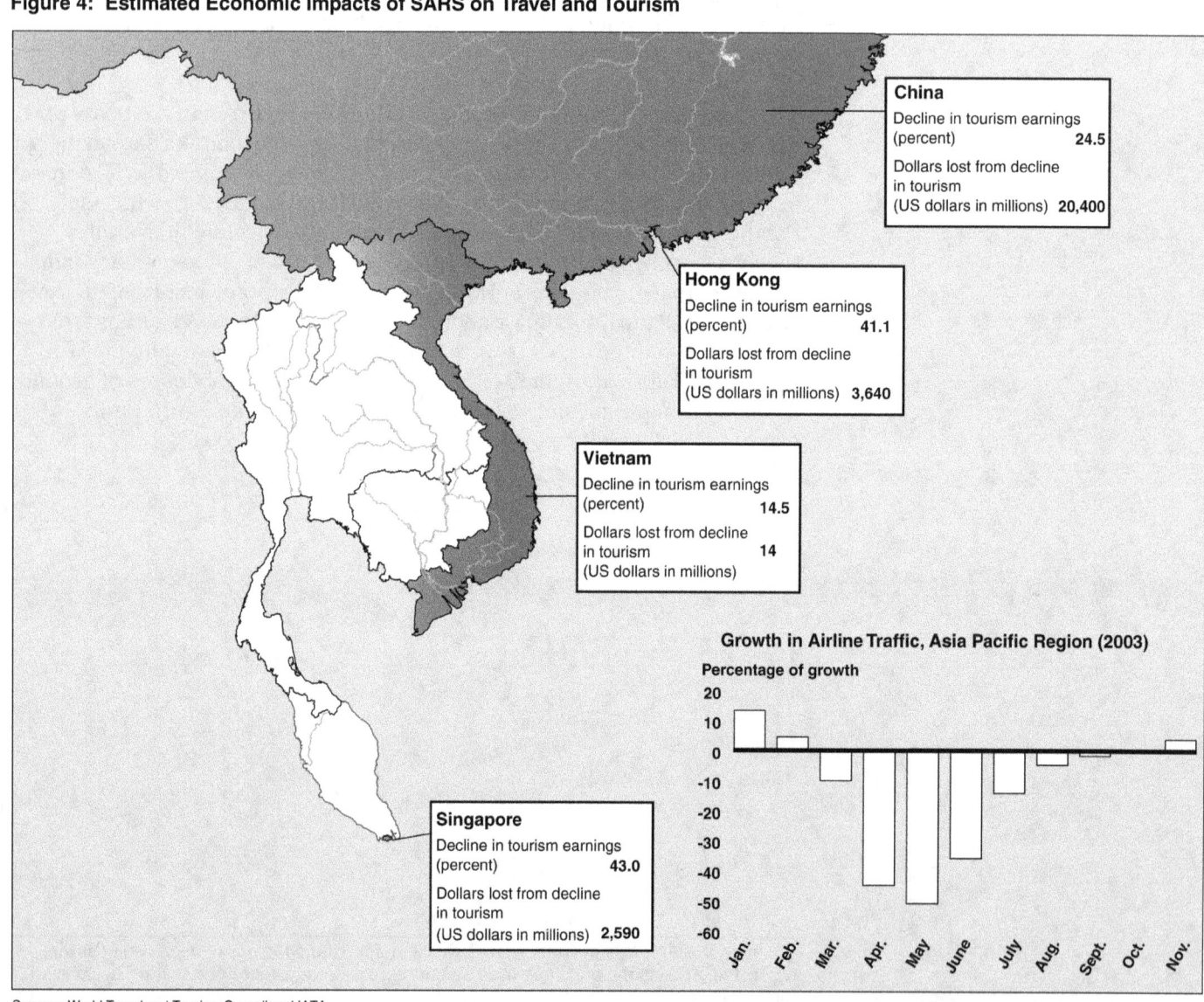

China
Decline in tourism earnings (percent) **24.5**
Dollars lost from decline in tourism (US dollars in millions) **20,400**

Hong Kong
Decline in tourism earnings (percent) **41.1**
Dollars lost from decline in tourism (US dollars in millions) **3,640**

Vietnam
Decline in tourism earnings (percent) **14.5**
Dollars lost from decline in tourism **14**
(US dollars in millions)

Singapore
Decline in tourism earnings (percent) **43.0**
Dollars lost from decline in tourism (US dollars in millions) **2,590**

Growth in Airline Traffic, Asia Pacific Region (2003)
Percentage of growth

Jan. Feb. Mar. Apr. May June July Aug. Sept. Oct. Nov.

Sources: World Travel and Tourism Council and IATA.

Dampened consumer confidence from SARS also had negative impacts on retail sales and foreign trade and investment, according to anecdotal evidence. The retail sector was negatively affected by the SARS outbreak as consumers curbed shopping trips and visits to restaurants in fear of contracting SARS. For example, China shortened the weeklong May Day celebration that it introduced in 1999 to stimulate private consumption. As shown in figure 5, retail sales fell concurrent with the SARS outbreak in China, Hong Kong, Singapore, and Taiwan, a decline particularly important for Hong Kong and Taiwan due to their large retail sectors. However, the rebound in consumer confidence is also illustrated by an increase in retail sales in the third quarter of 2003. Regarding foreign trade and investment, trends in these variables indicate less distinct SARS-related declines.[34] Nonetheless, there is some indication of the impact of SARS on these activities, such as the reduced sales at the major Guangzhou Trade Fair in China, which totaled only 26 percent of the previous year's amount, or the lagged effect of a decrease in foreign direct investment into China in July 2003.

---

[34]Foreign trade and investment were more resilient than consumption during the initial stages of the outbreak such that estimated economic effects were less significant due to the rapid rebound of Asian economies in the third quarter of 2003.

Figure 5: Quarterly Retail Sales Growth in Selected Asian Economies, 2002-2003

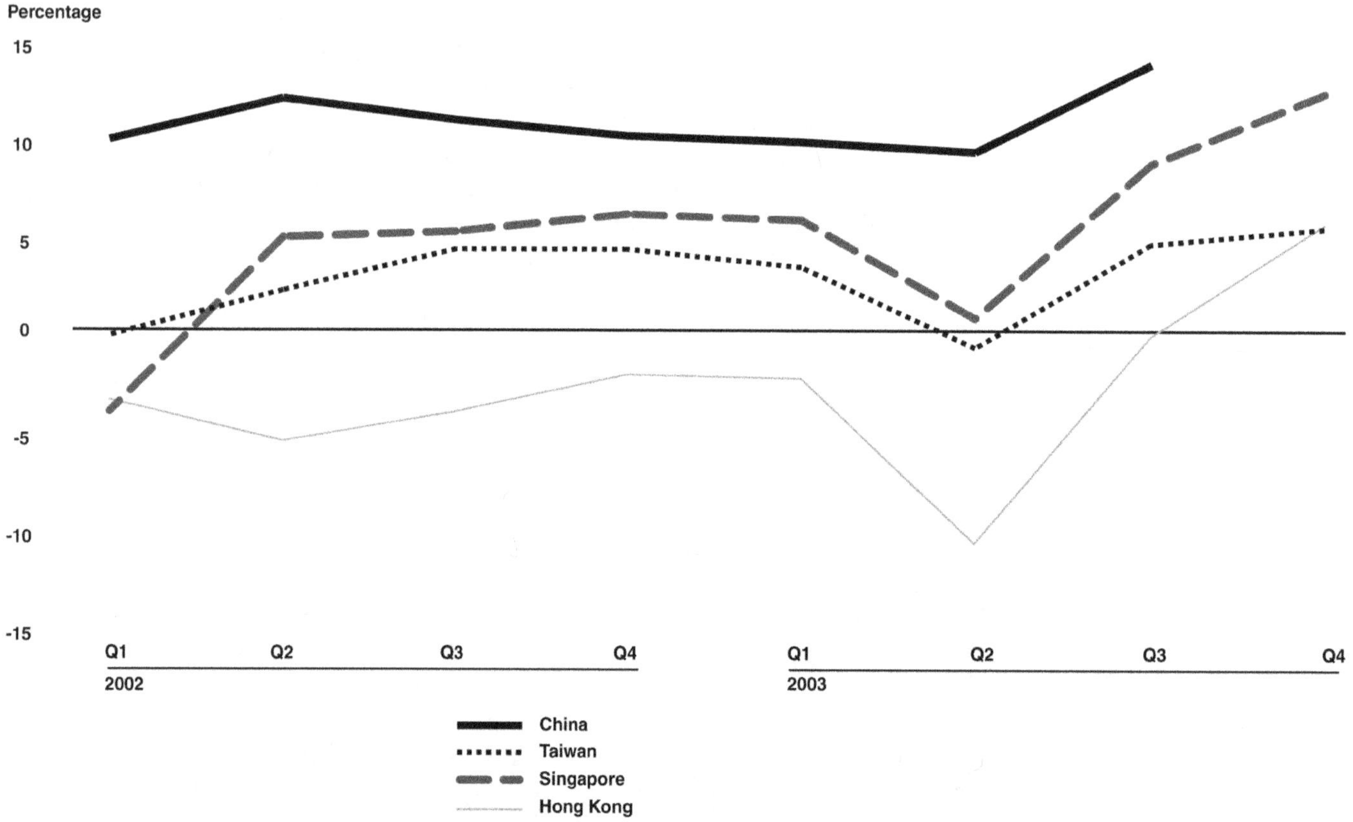

Percentage

Source: GAO analysis of data from national statistical offices in China, Hong Kong, Singapore, and Taiwan.

Asian Governments Provided Economic Stimulus Packages That Cost Billions

In response to SARS, governments in Asia implemented economic stimulus packages that also cost billions of dollars. Asian governments provided spending for medical and public health sectors to prevent and control the spread of SARS as well as for fiscal policy programs to more generally stimulate the economy. As shown in table 2, the Asian Development Bank estimates that the cost of these stimulus packages in the region could total nearly $9 billion. While many of the spending and tax measures are designed to improve GDP growth, they can also be considered an economic cost of SARS due to the diversion of government expenditures away from investments in needed public services.

Table 2: Asian Government Stimulus Packages in Response to SARS, 2003

(U.S. dollars in millions)

	Type of package	Cost of package
China	• Temporary tax relief and subsidies for affected industries • Free medical treatment for the poor and some price controls on SARS-related drugs and goods	3,500
Hong Kong	• Temporary tax relief, job creation, and loan guarantee schemes	1,500
Malaysia	• Loan programs, support for tourism-related industries, and job training	1,920
Singapore	• Temporary reduction in tourism and transport administrative fees, and relief measures for airlines	132
Taiwan	• Partial reimbursement of business-related losses for affected industries • Partial reimbursement for medical costs	1,400
Thailand	• General funding allocated as emergency budget	468

Source: GAO analysis of Asian Development Bank data.

WHO Members Will Debate Important Issues Raised by International Health Regulations' Revision

The SARS epidemic elevated the importance of the International Health Regulations' revision process. The proposed revisions, currently in draft form and scheduled for completion in May 2005, would expand the regulations' coverage and encourage better cooperation between member states and WHO. Member states will have to resolve at least five important issues, regarding (1) scope of coverage, (2) WHO's authority to conduct investigations in countries absent their consent, (3) the public health capacity of developing country members, (4) an enforcement mechanism to resolve compliance issues, and (5) how to ensure public health security without unnecessary interference with travel and trade.

Revisions Would Expand Coverage and Facilitate Cooperation, but Key Questions Remain

The draft regulations expand the scope of reporting beyond the current three diseases to include all events potentially constituting a public health emergency of international concern, such as SARS. They also promote enhanced member state cooperation with WHO and other countries. Additional changes under consideration include (1) designating national focal points with WHO for notification of public health emergencies and (2) requiring minimum core surveillance and response capacities at the national level to implement a global health security strategy. The overall goal of the revision process is to create a framework under which WHO and others can actively assist states in responding to international public health risks by directly linking the revised regulations to the work of GOARN.

Nevertheless, the draft regulations contain several provisions that have been the subject of ongoing debate, including:

- **Scope of coverage.** As part of the revision process, WHO has developed criteria to determine whether an outbreak is serious, unexpected, and likely to spread internationally. Furthermore, the draft regulations broaden the definition of a reportable disease to include significant illness caused by biological, chemical, or radionuclear sources. In its initial comments to WHO on the draft regulations, the U.S. government supported the use of criteria for determining what would be a public health emergency of international concern. Nevertheless, the U.S. strongly believed that the draft should also require reporting of a defined list of certain known, serious, communicable diseases that have the potential for creating such a concern.

- **Authority to conduct investigations.** Member states are considering the appropriate level of authority for the regulations. Specifically, an unresolved issue is the degree to which the regulations will require binding international commitments or more voluntary standards. To address this issue, member states are examining whether the benefits that would result from agreeing to more rigorous, comprehensive, and mandatory regulations would outweigh losses in sovereignty. For example, the draft regulations eliminate the language in the current regulations that specifically requires WHO to first obtain consent from the member state involved before conducting on-the-spot investigations of disease outbreaks.[35] However, the draft regulations are still somewhat ambiguous about whether consent is necessary.[36] According to a senior

---

[35]According to WHO officials, the language in the draft regulations dealing with conducting on-the-spot investigations was intended to closely reflect wording used in World Health Assembly Resolution 58.28, adopted on May 28, 2003, which among other things, urged WHO members to give high priority to IHR revision.

[36]For example, article 8(3) of the draft regulations states that "the health administration in whose territory the alleged event . . . is occurring **shall** collaborate with WHO in assessing the potential for international disease spread and possible interference with international traffic and the adequacy of control measures and, **when necessary**, in conducting on-the-spot studies by a team sent by WHO . . ." (emphasis added).

GAO-04-564 Emerging Infectious Diseases

WHO official, the proposed regulations were intentionally left vague about consent because it is a subject that members will want to debate thoroughly.

- **Public health capacity of developing countries.** The draft regulations provide member states with direction regarding the minimum core surveillance and response capacities required at the national level, including at airports, ports, and other points of entry. However, U.S. and WHO officials note that many developing countries currently lack even the most rudimentary public health capacity and will be dependent on significant international assistance to reach minimum surveillance and response capabilities. HHS officials have expressed caution about developing more comprehensive and demanding requirements that will be difficult for many countries with limited resources to implement. WHO officials acknowledge that, while WHO is able to provide technical assistance through GOARN, multilateral institutions, such as the World Bank, and donor countries will have to provide significant resources for developing countries to meet minimum surveillance and response requirements. A WHO official also indicated that while the proposed revisions to the regulations do not have specific provisions on technical assistance, developing countries are likely to raise the issue of adding such a provision during the revision process.

- **Enforcement mechanism.** The members will have to address what kind of enforcement mechanism they want included in the regulations to resolve compliance issues and to deal with violations of the regulations. According to WHO officials, failure to comply with WHO public health requirements is often a problem. The draft regulations, like the current regulations, include a nonbinding mechanism for resolving disputes. Thus, the WHO Director-General is directed either to (1) make every effort to resolve disputes or (2) refer disputes to a WHO Review Committee, which is tasked to forward its views and advice to the parties involved. Although WHO would continue to be dependent on the voluntary compliance of member states, WHO officials believe that if key countries (such as the United States) and neighboring trade partners are sufficiently concerned about the dangers of emerging diseases to press for compliance with the revised regulations, other countries are likely to fulfill their obligations. Furthermore, though it is too early to predict how China's response to SARS in 2003 will affect future compliance, WHO officials say the negative political, economic, and public health effects China suffered from its initial response to

SARS served as a warning to countries that ignore their international public health responsibilities.

- **International traffic.** The stated purpose of the draft regulations, which is similar to the current regulations, is to provide security against the international spread of disease while avoiding unnecessary interference with international traffic. Although the term international traffic appears to refer to international travel and trade, neither the proposed nor the current regulations define the term. Furthermore, the draft regulations do not include detailed criteria for determining what constitutes interference with international trade and travel.[37] A WHO official indicated that it was preferable not to include detailed criteria and to allow this issue to be decided on a case-by-case basis because of the very broad range of situations that could ultimately cause such interference. This issue could receive a good deal of attention in the revision process as member states try to balance medical and economic concerns. According to WHO officials, in past epidemics, concerns about economic loss and restrictions on trade and travel caused some countries not to report outbreaks within their borders and to refuse international assistance. Furthermore, for certain outbreaks—for example, those involving cholera in Peru in 1991 and plague in India in 1994—some experts reported that the international response may have exceeded the level of threat and led to unwarranted trade and travel losses in those countries.

Completing the Revision Process Seen as High Priority

The process for revising the International Health Regulations was intensified by a WHO World Health Assembly resolution passed in May 2003, during the SARS outbreak, urging members to give high priority to the revision process and to provide the resources and cooperation to facilitate this work.[38] The resolution also requested that the WHO Director-General consider informal sources of information to respond to outbreaks such as SARS; collaborate with national authorities in assessing the severity of infectious disease threats and the adequacy of control measures; and, when necessary, send a WHO team to conduct on-the-spot studies in places

---

[37]The draft regulations only state that "significant interference" is a "refusal of entry or departure or delaying entry or departure for more than 24 hours, for travelers and conveyances." WHO, Proposed International Health Regulations, art. 7.4.

[38]WHO, World Health Assembly Res. 56.28 (May 28, 2003).

experiencing infectious disease outbreaks. Although the resolution did not impose legally binding obligations on members, according to WHO officials and some observers it did lay the political groundwork for improved international cooperation on infectious disease control.

In January 2004, WHO distributed to its member states an interim draft of the revisions proposed by the WHO Secretariat. Composed of 55 articles and 10 technical annexes, the draft will be discussed in a series of regional consultations throughout 2004. The degree of consensus on the draft's technical and political issues will then determine the need for subsequent meetings at the global level. The goal is to convene an intergovernmental working group at the end of 2004 to finalize revisions to the draft regulations. It is hoped the regulations will then be ready for submission to the 58th World Health Assembly in May 2005. However, according to WHO and HHS officials, reaching both technical and political consensus on the regulations will be a difficult task, and they expect the revision process to extend beyond its target date.

Conclusion

While the 2002-2003 SARS outbreak had an impact on health and commerce in Asia, the extensive response by WHO and Asian governments, supported in large measure by the U.S. government, was ultimately effective in controlling the outbreak. This event highlighted a number of important issues, including the limited resources to support WHO's global infectious disease network and deficiencies in Asian governments' public health systems. It also revealed limitations in the International Health Regulations.

In the aftermath of SARS, WHO and member states have recognized the importance of strengthening international collaboration and cooperation to respond to global infectious disease outbreaks. To be successful, this effort will require a greater commitment of resources for global infectious disease control and a concerted effort to revise the International Health Regulations to make them more relevant and useful in future outbreaks. As the regulations are revised, WHO and member states face the challenge of improving the management of disease outbreaks while mitigating adverse economic impacts. The content, manner of acceptance, and means of enacting the final revisions are not certain, and much work remains to be done to resolve outstanding issues. As of April 2004, SARS has not re-emerged to cause another major international outbreak, but outbreaks of other infectious diseases can be expected in the future. Therefore, strengthening public health capacity will be essential for responding to future infectious disease outbreaks.

The SARS outbreak also revealed gaps in U.S. government protective measures, including difficulties in arranging medical evacuations from overseas and the inability to trace and contact individuals exposed to SARS during travel. In regard to tracing international travelers who may have been exposed to an infectious disease, we believe that amending HHS regulations to specify that the agency has authority to obtain this information would assist this effort. This action would facilitate HHS's ability to obtain necessary contact information (1) from airlines or shipping companies that may have concerns about sharing passenger information with HHS, or (2) in the event that issues involving coordination with other federal agencies cannot be effectively resolved.

Recommendations for Executive Action

This report is making three recommendations to improve the response to infectious disease outbreaks. First, to strengthen the international response, we recommend that the Secretary of Health and Human Services, in collaboration with the Secretary of State, work with WHO and official representatives from other WHO member states to strengthen WHO's global infectious disease network capacity to respond to disease outbreaks, for example, by expanding the available pool of public health experts.

Second, to help Health and Human Services prevent the introduction, transmission, or spread of infectious diseases into the United States, we recommend that the Secretary of HHS complete the necessary steps to ensure that the agency can obtain passenger contact information in a timely and comprehensive manner, including, if necessary, the promulgation of regulations specifically for this purpose.

Third, to protect U.S. government employees and their families working overseas and to better support other U.S. citizens living or traveling overseas, we recommend that the Secretary of State continue to work with the Secretaries of Health and Human Services and Defense to identify public and private sector resources for medical evacuations during infectious disease outbreaks and develop procedures for arranging these evacuations. Such efforts could include

- working with private air ambulance companies and the Department of Defense to determine their capacity for transporting patients with an emerging infectious disease such as SARS, and

- working to develop agreements under which U.S. medical facilities near international ports of entry will accept medically evacuated patients with infectious diseases such as SARS.

Agency Comments and Our Evaluation

HHS, State, and WHO provided written comments on a draft of this report (see apps. IV, V, and VI for a reprint of HHS's, State's, and WHO's comments). They also provided technical and clarifying comments that we have incorporated where appropriate. HHS said the report is a good summary of the SARS outbreak in Asia and the actions taken by WHO, affected countries, and U.S. agencies. HHS stated that the report's recommendations are appropriate and emphasized the national and international interagency collaboration that will be required to implement them in preparation for the next epidemic. HHS also noted that to carry out some of the recommendations, sensitive legal and privacy issues and diplomatic concerns must be carefully addressed. HHS also noted that the report contains a useful overview of WHO's efforts to revise its International Health Regulations and correctly ties WHO's increased effort to the impact of SARS and lessons learned. In that regard, HHS provided additional information on coordination and collaboration efforts it took during the outbreak.

State indicated that the report is a useful summary of the SARS outbreak and its impact and documents important lessons for other infectious disease outbreaks beyond the 2003 SARS epidemic. Regarding our first recommendation, State said it is committed to working with WHO and its member states to strengthen the response capacity of WHO's global infectious disease network. Regarding our recommendation on contact tracing of arriving passengers infected or exposed to infectious disease, State noted that it has been working on this issue with its interagency partners since the SARS outbreak but underscored that serious legal issues still exist for both the United States and other governments. State also agreed with our recommendation on developing procedures for arranging medical evacuations during an airborne infectious disease outbreak. State indicated that it is working with CDC to develop protocols on how to handle medical evacuations for quarantinable diseases but noted that capacity for such medical evacuations will be limited, as will capacity of U.S. medical facilities to handle a large influx of patients.

WHO stated that, overall, the report provides a factual analysis of the events surrounding the emergence of SARS and addresses the major weaknesses in national and international control efforts. WHO noted, however, that the report presents major criticisms of the response by China, Hong Kong, and Taiwan to SARS but does not reflect these governments' actions throughout the SARS epidemic or the depth and intensity of their control efforts later on. WHO also stated that the report puts little emphasis on other countries that experienced problems— Canada, for example. We disagree that the report does not adequately balance the governments' shortcomings with accomplishments, as the report includes specific sections on improved screening and reporting of SARS cases, rapid isolation and contact tracing, enhanced hospital infection control practices, and quarantine measures. The report details steps Asian governments have taken in response to SARS to build capacity for future outbreaks. The preponderance of our evidence on Asian governments' response was provided directly by Chinese, Hong Kong, and Taiwan government and public health officials and from post-SARS evaluation reports produced by these governments and WHO-sponsored conferences. We focused our report on the response of China, Hong Kong, and Taiwan since 95 percent of the SARS cases occurred there. The response of other countries, such as Canada was outside the scope of our examination.

Regarding our discussion of WHO's global infectious disease network, WHO stated that GOARN is one of the mechanisms by which WHO mobilizes technical resources for outbreak investigation and response provided further information about the role of the Western Pacific Regional Office (WPRO) in the SARS response. We clarified the role of GOARN and expanded our discussion on the activities of WPRO. WHO also said that its response was challenged, but not constrained, by limited resources. While we agree with this more general characterization, we believe that not being able to obtain the appropriate multidisciplinary staff and sustain a response over time were significant constraints that warrant serious attention in preparing for future emerging infectious diseases. WHO also noted that the world's dependence on a fragile process and on the personal commitment and sacrifice of WHO and GOARN staff is a concern.

Scope and Methodology

To assess WHO's actions to respond to SARS in Asia, we analyzed WHO policy, program, and budget documents, including WHO's Web-based situation updates and guidelines that served as the primary instrument for disseminating information on SARS. We interviewed WHO officials responsible for managing the international response at WHO headquarters in Geneva and public health specialists who served on country teams that were deployed to Asia. We examined WHO's GOARN, including its guiding principles and how it operated during the SARS outbreak. We also interviewed Asian government officials in Beijing, Guangdong Province, Hong Kong, and Taipei who received WHO's technical advice and support; U.S. government officials; and recognized experts within the public health community.

To assess the role of the U.S. government in responding to SARS in Asia and limiting its spread into the United States, we analyzed program documents and interviewed officials from the Departments of Health and Human Services, State, Defense, and Homeland Security, and the U.S. Centers for Disease Control and Prevention (CDC). To examine CDC's ability to trace travelers who may have been exposed to an infectious disease, we interviewed officials from the Air Transport Association and the Department of Transportation and reviewed applicable legislation and regulations. To assess State's ability to provide medical evacuation of U.S. citizens, we examined CDC guidelines on air transport of SARS patients and interviewed officials from major private medical evacuation companies. We also interviewed U.S. embassy (Beijing), consulate (Hong Kong and Guangzhou), and American Institute in Taiwan officials responsible for managing the U.S. government response at the country level.

To describe how governments in Asia responded to the SARS outbreak, we focused on those parts of Asia most affected by SARS in the 2002-2003 outbreak, including China, Hong Kong, and Taiwan. While in the region, we met with public health officials at various levels responsible for managing their governments' public health response, including senior ministry of health and provincial and municipal government officials, as well as hospital administrators and health care workers. We also examined government documents on public health programs and post-SARS evaluations, and reviewed applicable China, Hong Kong, and Taiwan laws and regulations.

To describe the economic impact of SARS in Asia, we reviewed impact estimates provided by (1) the Asian Development Bank's Economic and Research Department, which used a simulation model from Oxford Economic Forecasting; (2) a simulation model using data from the Global

Trade Analysis Project Consortium;[39] and (3) a simulation model by Global Insight, a leading U.S. economic data and forecasting firm. Specifics of each of these models are discussed in appendix III. Another organization, the *Far Eastern Economic Review*, a regional economic business weekly, gathered studies and data on SARS and reported a summary cost estimate that we also reviewed. To supplement our analysis of these impact estimates, we examined trends in official macroeconomic data as reported by the countries' central banks or departments of statistics, the Asian Development Bank, the Organization for Economic Cooperation and Development, and the World Travel and Tourism Association.[40] Trends in international airline traffic were obtained from the International Air Transport Association. We corroborated our findings with information provided by the U.S. National Intelligence Council and interviews with government officials in Asia.

Finally, to examine the status of efforts to update the International Health Regulations, we reviewed the current International Health Regulations, a draft of WHO's proposed revision of the regulations, the initial U.S. government response to the proposed revisions, and the WHO constitution. We also interviewed WHO and U.S. government officials who are actively engaged in the revision process and other legal experts to determine the potential impacts of the revised rules.

We performed our work from July 2003 to April 2004 in accordance with generally accepted government auditing standards.

We are sending copies of this report to the Secretaries of Health and Human Services, State, and Defense; appropriate congressional committees; and other interested parties. We will also make copies available to others upon request. In addition, the report will be available at no charge on GAO's Web site at http://www.gao.gov.

---

[39]Jong-Wha Lee and Warwick J. McKibbon, "Globalization and Disease: The Case of SARS, Working Paper No. 2003/16," Research School of Pacific and Asian Studies, Australian National University and the Brookings Institution, Washington, D.C. (2003).

[40]To determine the reliability of the official national accounts data, we verified that the general patterns reported were consistent with other documentary evidence and reviewed each economy's compliance with the International Monetary Fund's data dissemination standards. We conclude that the data is sufficiently reliable for the purposes of establishing decreased economic activity during the second quarter of 2003.

If you or your staff have any questions, please contact one of us. Other contacts and key contributors are listed in appendix VII.

Sincerely yours,

David Gootnick
Director, International Affairs and Trade

Janet Heinrich
Director, Health Care—Public Health Issues

SARS Cases and Deaths, November 2002–July 2003

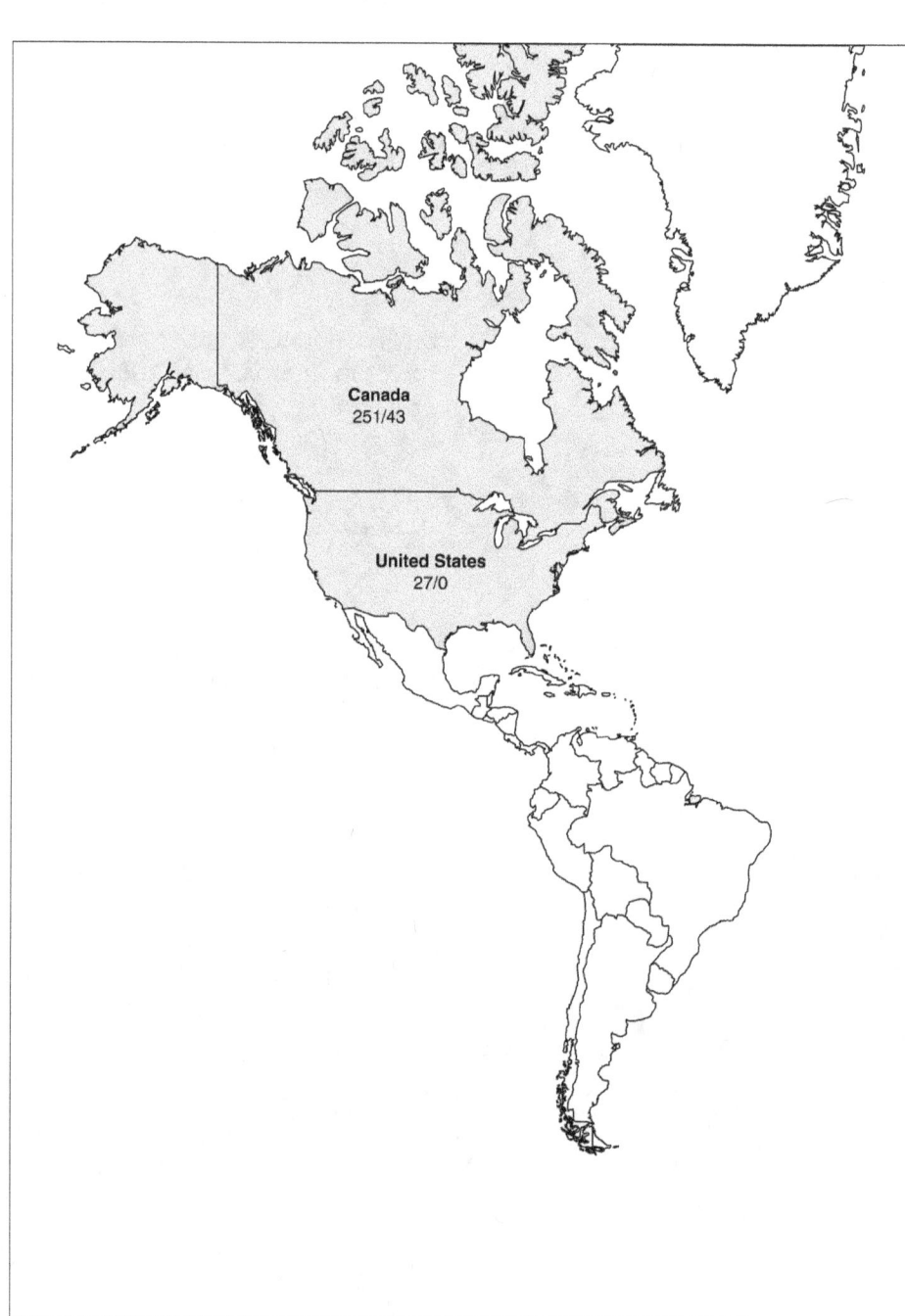

Canada
251/43

United States
27/0

Sources: World Health Organization and CDC.

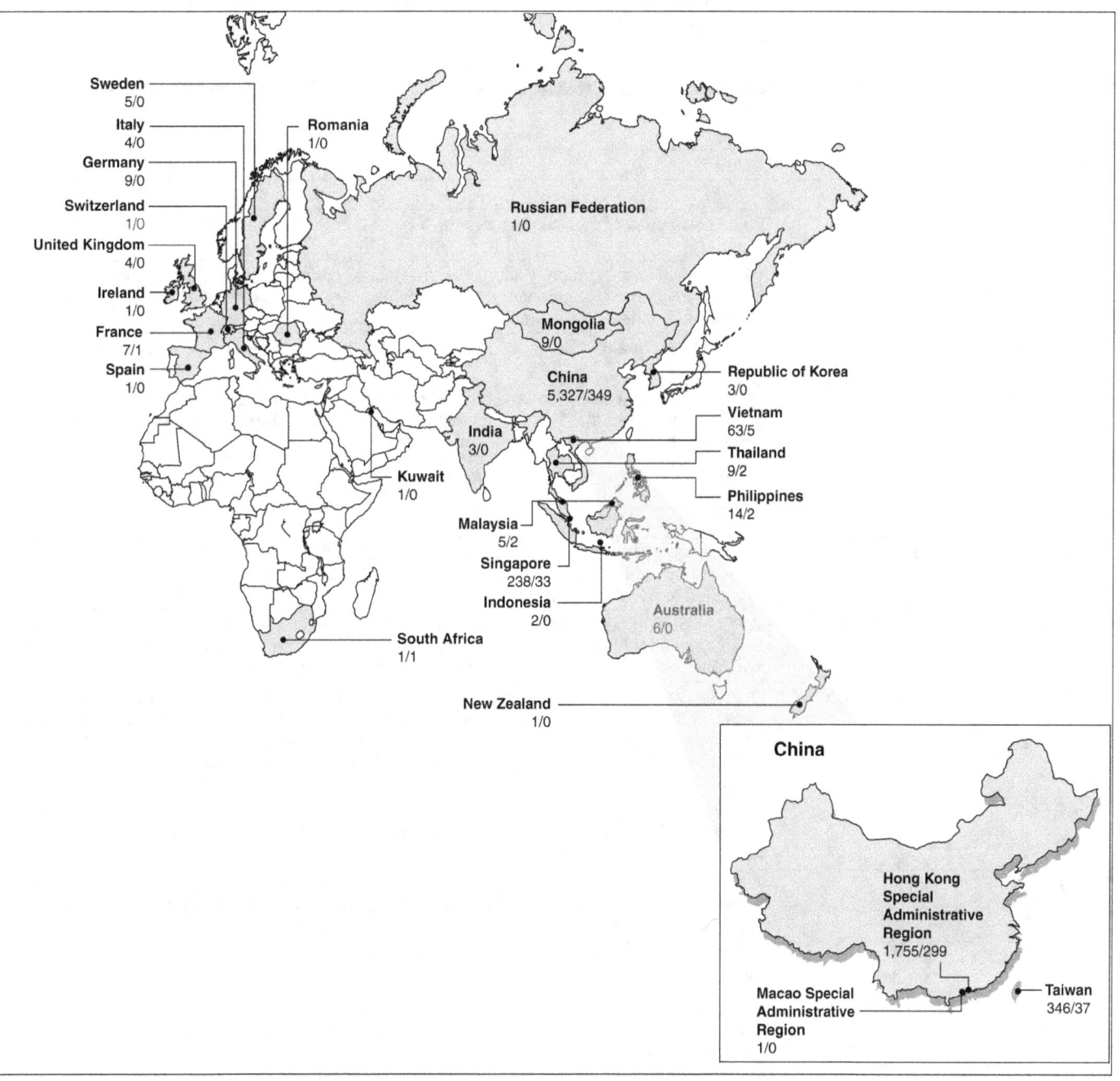

Sweden
5/0

Italy
4/0

Germany
9/0

Switzerland
1/0

United Kingdom
4/0

Ireland
1/0

France
7/1

Spain
1/0

Romania
1/0

Russian Federation
1/0

Mongolia
9/0

China
5,327/349

India
3/0

Kuwait
1/0

Malaysia
5/2

Singapore
238/33

Indonesia
2/0

South Africa
1/1

New Zealand
1/0

Republic of Korea
3/0

Vietnam
63/5

Thailand
9/2

Philippines
14/2

Australia
6/0

China

Hong Kong
Special
Administrative
Region
1,755/299

Macao Special
Administrative
Region
1/0

Taiwan
346/37

Note: Numbers represent cases and deaths.

SARS Chronology

Appendix II lists key worldwide events during the SARS outbreak, from November 2002, when the disease first emerged, to the most recent reported cases in January 2004.

Year	Location	Event
2002		
November 16	Guangdong Province, China[a]	First known case of atypical pneumonia, later determined to be SARS.
November 23	Beijing	World Health Organization (WHO) influenza expert attends workshop in Beijing and learns from a participant from Guangdong Province of a "serious outbreak with high mortality and involvement of health care staff."
November 27	Canada	Global Public Health Intelligence Network (GPHIN) picks up reports of a "flu outbreak" in China.
Mid-December	WHO Headquarters, Geneva	WHO requests further information from China on the influenza outbreak. Chinese government replies that influenza activity in Beijing and Guangdong is normal and that surveillance system detected no unusual strains of the virus.
December 10	Guangdong Province	Infection in second city in Guangdong Province.
2003		
January 23	Guangdong Province	Guangdong's provincial health authorities produce a report about the outbreak detailing the nature of transmission, clinical features, and suggested preventive measures. The report is circulated to hospitals in the province, but is not shared with WHO or Hong Kong.
February 10-11	Multiple Locations	WHO Beijing office, Global Outbreak and Alert Response Network (GOARN) partners, and U.S. Centers for Disease Control (CDC) receive reports of a "strange contagious disease" and "pneumonic plague" causing deaths in Guangdong Province.
February 14-20	China, Hong Kong	Chinese Center for Disease Control and Prevention erroneously announces that the probable causative agent of the atypical pneumonia is *Chlamydia*. At the same time, cases of avian influenza in a family that traveled between Hong Kong and China result in two deaths. This leads to speculation that the atypical pneumonia outbreak is caused by avian influenza. WHO activates its global influenza laboratory network and calls for heightened global surveillance.
February 21	Hong Kong[a]	First superspreader event in Hong Kong: A physician from Guangdong Province stays at the Metropole Hotel in Hong Kong and is soon hospitalized with respiratory failure. While at the hotel, he transmits the disease to at least 16 other people.
February 23	China	A team of WHO experts, including CDC staff, arrives in Beijing but is given limited access to information; Chinese authorities deny WHO's repeated requests for permission to travel to Guangdong Province.
February 24	WHO Headquarters, Geneva	GPHIN detects Chinese newspaper report that more than 50 hospital staff in Guangzhou are infected with "mysterious pneumonia."
February 26	Vietnam[a]	Chinese-American businessman admitted to the French Hospital in Hanoi with fever and respiratory symptoms.

(Continued From Previous Page)

Year	Location	Event
February 28	Vietnam	WHO official Dr. Carlo Urbani notifies WHO office in Manila of an unusual disease. WHO headquarters moves to heightened state of alert.
Early March	United States	State Department establishes an intradepartmental working group to deal with impact of outbreak.
March 1	Singapore[a]	Woman who stayed at the Metropole Hotel in Hong Kong is hospitalized with respiratory symptoms.
March 4	Hong Kong	Second superspreader event in Hong Kong: a resident who had visited the Metropole Hotel is admitted to hospital with respiratory symptoms; within a week, at least 25 hospital staff, all linked to the patient's ward, develop respiratory illness.
March 5	Canada[a]	Toronto woman who also stayed at the Metropole Hotel in Hong Kong dies at home. Shortly after, her son becomes ill, is admitted to Scarborough Grace Hospital, and dies. His admission triggers an outbreak at the hospital.
March 8	Taiwan[a]	Businessman with travel history to Guangdong Province is hospitalized with respiratory symptoms.
March 10	China	Chinese Health Ministry asks WHO for technical and laboratory support to clarify cause of the Guangdong outbreak of atypical pneumonia.
March 12	WHO Headquarters, Geneva	WHO issues global alert about cases of severe atypical pneumonia following mounting reports of spread among hospital staff in Hong Kong and Hanoi. CDC offers assistance to WHO.
March 13	WHO Headquarters, Geneva	WHO sends emergency alert to GOARN partners.
March 14	United States	CDC activates Emergency Operations Center.
March 15	WHO Headquarters, Geneva	WHO issues rare global travel advisory, names the mysterious illness "severe acute respiratory syndrome" (SARS), and declares it a "worldwide health threat." WHO issues its first definitions of suspect and probable cases, calls on travelers to be aware of symptoms, and issues advice to airlines.
March 15	United States[a]	CDC issues travel advisory suggesting postponement of nonessential travel to Hong Kong, Guangdong Province, and Hanoi. CDC issues preliminary case definition for suspected SARS and initiates domestic surveillance for SARS. First suspected U.S. case is identified.
March 16	United States	CDC begins distributing health alert cards to passengers arriving from Hong Kong at four international airports.
Mid-March	Taiwan	CDC team arrives in Taiwan to assist in SARS response.
March 17	WHO Headquarters, Geneva, and multiple locations	WHO sets up worldwide network of laboratories to expedite detection of causative agent and to develop a robust and reliable diagnostic test. A similar network is set up to pool clinical knowledge on symptoms, diagnosis, and management. A third network is set up to study SARS epidemiology.
March 28	China	China joins WHO's collaborative networks, initially set up on March 17.
March 30	Hong Kong	Third superspreader event in Hong Kong: Health authorities announce that 213 residents of Amoy Gardens housing estate have been hospitalized with SARS.
April 2	WHO Headquarters, Geneva	WHO issues most stringent travel advisory in its 55-year history, recommending that people postpone all but essential travel to Hong Kong and Guangdong Province until further notice.
April 3	China	WHO team arrives in Guangdong.

(Continued From Previous Page)

Year	Location	Event
April 4	United States	President Bush signs executive order adding SARS to the list of quarantinable communicable diseases. This order provides CDC, through its Division of Global Migration and Quarantine, with the legal authority to implement isolation and quarantine measures.
April 16	WHO Headquarters, Geneva	WHO laboratory network announces conclusive identification of SARS causative agent: a new coronavirus.
April 19-20	China	Change in political stance by Chinese leadership. Top leaders advise officials not to cover up cases of SARS; mayor of Beijing and Health Minister, both of whom downplayed the SARS threat, are removed from their posts.
April 28	Vietnam	First country to successfully contain its outbreak of SARS.
May 2	United States	State Department holds interagency meeting on SARS.
May 3	Taiwan	WHO sends officials to Taiwan to assist CDC team.
May 17	WHO Headquarters, Geneva	First global consultation on SARS epidemiology concludes its work, confirming that available evidence supports the control measures recommended by WHO.
May 27	WHO Headquarters, Geneva	World Health Assembly resolution recognizes the severity of the threat that SARS poses and calls on all countries to report cases promptly and transparently. A second resolution strengthens WHO's capacity to respond to disease outbreaks.
June 17-18	Malaysia	WHO holds Global Conference on SARS to review scientific findings on SARS and examine public health interventions to contain it.
July 5	WHO Headquarters, Geneva	WHO announces that the global SARS outbreak has been contained.
September 8	Singapore	Singapore announces that a medical researcher is infected with SARS. Based on an investigation of this incident, WHO concludes that the patient was accidentally infected in the laboratory.
December 17	Taiwan	Taiwan announces that a researcher is infected with SARS. Public health authorities conclude that the infection was acquired in a laboratory.
December 20-January 5, 2004	China	A man in Guangdong Province is hospitalized with SARS-like symptoms on December 20. Chinese authorities inform WHO on December 26. After initial diagnostic tests are inconclusive, authorities send the samples to two WHO-designated reference laboratories in Hong Kong. On January 5, the laboratories confirm that the patient has SARS. None of the patient's contacts contracted SARS.
December 31-January 17, 2004	China	A woman in Guangdong Province is hospitalized with SARS-like symptoms on December 31. Chinese authorities inform WHO and samples are submitted to two WHO-designated reference laboratories in Hong Kong. On January 17, Chinese authorities announce that the patient has SARS. None of the patient's contacts contracted SARS.
2004		
January 6-27	China	A man in Guangdong Province is hospitalized with SARS-like symptoms on January 6. Chinese authorities inform WHO and samples are submitted to WHO-designated reference laboratories in Hong Kong. On January 27, WHO announces that the patient has probable SARS.

(Continued From Previous Page)

Year	Location	Event
January 7-30	China	A doctor in Guangdong Province becomes ill with SARS-like symptoms and is diagnosed with pneumonia on January 14. However, he was not properly isolated in hospital until January 16, he was not declared as a suspected SARS case to China's Ministry of Health until January 26, and WHO was not informed until January 30.
January 9-16	China	A team of international experts from WHO conducts a joint investigative mission in Guangdong Province with colleagues from China's Ministry of Health, Ministry of Agriculture, the Chinese Center for Disease Control and Prevention, and the Guangdong Center for Disease Control and Prevention to identify the sources of infection of the most recent SARS cases. The team finds no definitive source of infection for any of the cases.

Source: GAO analysis of WHO and CDC data.

[a]Date of the first known case(s) of SARS.

Estimates of the Economic Impact of SARS

Estimates of the economic impact of SARS have been produced by multiple sources and vary due to the inexact nature of estimating the impact of a recent event such as SARS. When the SARS outbreak first emerged, a number of institutions began estimating the potential economic impact of the disease. These institutions included private investment banks, industry organizations, academics, consulting firms, and international financial institutions such as the Asian Development Bank. To produce their estimates, assumptions had to be incorporated regarding the expected duration of SARS, the number of sectors affected, and country-specific macroeconomic conditions. As such, estimates of economic impact have been broad in nature, have varied depending on model assumptions, and were often revised when actual data were received. For example, some of the initial economic impact estimates were revised downward once data emerged showing China's strong economic growth during the first 4 months of 2003.

To describe the economic impact of SARS in Asia, we primarily relied on impact estimates generated from institutions using simulation models. Table 3 provides information on the models we reviewed. As the table shows, each of these models was used to analyze a low scenario case and a high scenario case, which differed based on assumptions regarding the expected duration of the SARS outbreak and hence the expected duration of the shock to the economy resulting from SARS. To accord with the shorter duration of the actual outbreak, the low scenario results estimated the economic impact of SARS at roughly 0.5 percent to 2 percent of gross domestic product (GDP).[1] All three models show that the largest economic impacts as a percentage of GDP were estimated for Hong Kong and Singapore, which is due to their previously lowered consumption demand and high share of tourism and retail.

---

[1]The International Monetary Fund announced in April 2003 that the estimated decline in GDP due to SARS was 0.2 percent for China and 0.4 percent for East Asia. The World Bank's East Asia Update in April 2003 also provided an estimate of the decline in GDP due to SARS at 0.3 percent for East Asia. However, neither organization has published a model to describe how it arrived at these estimates.

Table 3: Models Estimating the Economic Impact of SARS on GDP in Asia, 2003

Source	Model description	Key assumptions	Country	Estimated decline in GDP (percentage)	
				Low scenario	High scenario
Asian Development Bank: May 2003 ERD Policy Brief No. 15	Simulation model from the Oxford Economic Forecasting consulting firm	Low scenario: SARS shock lasts through second quarter of 2003 High scenario: SARS shock extends into third quarter of 2003	China Hong Kong Malaysia Singapore Taiwan Thailand	0.2 1.8 0.6 1.1 0.9 0.7	0.5 4.0 1.5 2.3 1.9 1.6
Jong-Wha Lee and Warwick McKibbin: "Globalization and Disease: The Case of SARS," Working Paper No. 2003/16, Research School of Pacific and Asian Studies, Australian National University and the Brookings Institution, Washington, D.C. (2003)	"G-Cubed" Asia Pacific world macroeconomic simulation model based on data from the Global Trade Analysis Project Consortium	Low scenario: SARS shock occurs in 2003 High scenario: SARS shock reoccurs after 2003 and fades over 10 years • SARS shock hits China and Hong Kong and affects other countries based on trade and tourist flows • SARS shock in 2003 lasts 6 months • Country risk premium increases by 200 basis points • Output falls by 15 percent and costs rise by 5 percent in affected service sectors	China Hong Kong Malaysia Singapore Taiwan Thailand	1.1 2.6 0.2 0.5 0.5 0.2	2.3 3.2 0.2 0.5 0.5 0.2
Global Insight: May 2003 Executive Summary of Asia and Oceania, "SARS Epidemic's Economic Impact on Asia"	In-house simulation model	Low scenario: SARS shock lasts through second quarter of 2003 High scenario: SARS shock extends to the end of 2003	China Hong Kong Malaysia Singapore Taiwan Thailand Vietnam	1.0 1.4 0.3 1.2 0.8 0.7 0.1	1.9 2.2 1.4 1.8 1.7 1.6 0.8

Source: GAO analysis of studies from the Asian Development Bank, Brookings Institution, and Global Insight.

In addition to the model estimates provided in table 3, we also reviewed SARS cost estimates provided by the *Far Eastern Economic Review*. The *Far Eastern Economic Review*'s estimate of $11 billion was generated by calculating an average estimated percentage loss in GDP using reports

from various governments and financial institutions and applying that
average to the nominal GDP figures provided by the International Monetary
Fund.[2]

---

[2]The *Far Eastern Economic Review* is a regional economic business weekly. Its cost
estimates of SARS are provided in a 2003 special report on the SARS outbreak. The financial
institutions that provided economic impact estimates to the review included Merrill Lynch,
Goldman Sachs, JP Morgan, Lehman Brothers, Morgan Stanley, ING Financial Markets, BNP
Paribas Peregrine, Standard & Poor's, and IDEAGlobal.

Comments from the Department of Health and Human Services

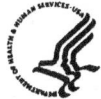

DEPARTMENT OF HEALTH & HUMAN SERVICES

Office of Inspector General

Washington, D.C. 20201

APR 1 6 2004

Mr. David Gootnick
Director, International Affairs and Trade
United States General Accounting Office
Washington, D.C. 20548

Dear Mr. Gootnick:

Enclosed are the Department's comments on your draft report entitled, "Emerging Infectious Diseases: Asian SARS Outbreak Challenged International and National Responses" (GAO-04-564). The comments represent the tentative position of the Department and are subject to reevaluation when the final version of this report is received.

The Department provided several technical comments directly to your staff.

The Department appreciates the opportunity to comment on this draft report before its publication.

Sincerely,

Dara Corrigan
Acting Principal Deputy Inspector General

Enclosure

The Office of Inspector General (OIG) is transmitting the Department's response to this draft report in our capacity as the Department's designated focal point and coordinator for General Accounting Office reports. OIG has not conducted an independent assessment of these comments and therefore expresses no opinion on them.

**COMMENTS OF THE DEPARTMENT OF HEALTH AND HUMAN SERVICES
ON THE GENERAL ACCOUNTING OFFICE'S DRAFT REPORT: "EMERGING
INFECTIOUS DISEASES: ASIAN SARS OUTBREAK CHALLENGED
INTERNATIONAL AND NATIONAL RESPONSES" (GAO-04-564)**

The report is a good summary of the Severe Acute Respiratory Syndrome (SARS)
outbreak in Southeast Asia and actions taken during and after the epidemic by the World
Health Organization (WHO) and the affected countries, as well as actions taken by the
Department of Health and Human Services (HHS) to combat the epidemic globally and to
protect the United States (U.S.), focusing on the activities of our Centers for Disease
Control and Prevention (CDC). The report also contains a useful overview of WHO's
efforts to revise its International Health Regulations and correctly ties the newly intense
efforts at WHO to the impact of SARS and lessons learned.

The SARS outbreak did indeed challenge international and national responses. While the
report correctly focuses on the issues and events, the intensity of the coordination and
collaboration within governments and among nations was unprecedented. The report
documents many of the activities, but does not go into detail on the substantial
coordination and collaboration efforts among U.S. executive branch agencies and among
those agencies and the governments in East and Southeast Asia. While we recognize the
latter was not the focus of this report, the following briefly describes how HHS organized
itself to manage its response and effectively faced the new challenges.

Tommy G. Thompson, as Secretary of HHS, led the Department's response to the SARS
epidemic, thus ensuring coordinated roles and responses across our agencies most directly
involved in the response domestically and internationally – CDC, the National Institutes
of Health, and the Food and Drug Administration. Primarily through his Office of Global
Health Affairs and Office of Public Health Emergency Preparedness, the Secretary also
provided the leadership to ensure the necessary coordination and alignment of our
domestic and international responses. Using the cutting-edge technology of his new
Command Center and face-to-face opportunities in Geneva and Washington, the Secretary
maintained close contact with the leadership at WHO and with a number of affected
governments, including Canada, the People's Republic of China, the Socialist Republic of
Vietnam, and the Hong Kong Special Administrative Region.

For example, after the 2003 SARS outbreak, China's Ministry of Health committed to
more open communication with HHS in any future avian influenza outbreak and to the
sharing with HHS of key laboratory samples from a localized SARS outbreak in
Guangdong that occurred last winter. Secretary Thompson also pledged to assist China in
its fight against SARS and other emerging diseases through collaboration of HHS
scientists working with their Chinese counterparts. The signing of this U.S.- China
Emerging Infections Program in May 2004 represents a multi-year, multi-million dollar
program of cooperation between HHS and the Chinese Ministry of Health aimed at
strengthening fundamental public health infrastructure and improving the national
capacity to manage a number of infectious diseases, including SARS and pandemic

1

influenza as part of a worldwide early warning surveillance network HHS is building. These are but a few examples of how Secretary Thompson's diplomatic efforts and leadership, in coordination with the Department of State (DOS), helped to obtain needed information for HHS and DOS about the global response and the collective and individual SARS efforts and challenges at the country-level. With assistance from DOS, Secretary Thompson's personal interventions and diplomatic outreach with Southeast Asian government counterparts substantially aided in gaining access to those countries by WHO and our own experts.

The Secretary and his senior staff used the Secretary's Command Center to hold daily briefings during which a CDC official, usually the Director, presented the latest information on the SARS situation worldwide and actions being taken overseas and domestically to protect the U.S. Experts from DOS, Homeland Security, and Defense participated in these briefings. Issues included coordination with WHO and affected countries, plans for scientific research, communication with the public, and communication with other national governments and economies, etc. Daily reports and maps, prepared by the Secretary's Command Center staff, facilitated the tracking of the epidemic and maximized the deployment of HHS staff.

HHS believes the increased inter-agency coordination and lessons we learned during the SARS epidemic in 2003 were highly useful in our response to the Avian Influenza (H5N1) outbreak in Asia in 2004. The interagency group has made progress on a number of international operational and policy issues since the Spring of 2003, and shaped our engagement in the process to revise the WHO International Health Regulations.

HHS believes this report makes a valuable contribution, and we find its recommendations to be appropriate. They identify important work that needs to be undertaken or brought to conclusion as quickly as possible so that we are sufficiently prepared for the next epidemic. The recommendations stress the interagency nature of the work to be done internationally as well as domestically. Again, the report correctly recognizes the importance of collaboration with our partner agencies, in particular the valuable interagency coordination activities under the purview of DOS. To carry out some of the recommendations, sensitive legal and privacy issues and diplomatic concerns must be carefully addressed.

2

Comments from the Department of State

United States Department of State

Assistant Secretary and Chief Financial Officer

Washington, D.C. 20520

APR 15 2004

Dear Ms. Williams-Bridgers:

    We appreciate the opportunity to review your draft report, "EMERGING INFECTIOUS DISEASES: Asian SARS Outbreak Challenged International and National Responses," GAO-04-564, GAO Job Code 320198.

    The enclosed Department of State comments are provided for incorporation with this letter as an appendix to the final report.

    If you have any questions concerning this response, please contact Sara Allinder Mestre, Foreign Affairs Officer, Bureau of Oceans and International Environment and Scientific Affairs, at (202) 647-3649.

Sincerely,

Christopher B. Burnham

cc: GAO – Patrick Dickriede
        OES – Lee Morin
        State/OIG – Mark Duda
        State/H – Paul Kelly

Department of State Comments on GAO Draft Report
EMERGING INFECTIOUS DISEASES: Asian SARS Outbreak Challenged
International and National Responses
(GAO-04-564, GAO Job Code 320198)

We appreciate the opportunity to comment on your draft report, "Emerging Infectious Diseases, Asian SARS Outbreak Challenged International and National Responses". The report is a useful summary of the Severe Acute Respiratory Syndrome (SARS) outbreak and its impact.

The Department of State agrees that the Asian SARS outbreak challenged international and national responses. At the outset, some Asian governments did not recognize the SARS emergency. The Department of State applied diplomatic pressure on governments to increase transparency and response, helped facilitate the U.S. government response to SARS in Asia, and provided information on SARS to U.S. government employees and citizens in the region. By the end of the outbreak in July 2003, SARS had served to heighten awareness of the need for surveillance and response activities and changed how nations think about reporting disease outbreaks internationally and internally. Both the World Health Organization (WHO) and its member states gained real-world insights that have benefited the process, under WHO auspices, of revising the International Health Regulations. The report correctly identifies the challenges in such a revision, but the fact that countries accept the need is a positive step forward.

The SARS outbreak also led to increasing coordination among Federal agencies charged with a response, and thus provided lessons learned, including for the Avian Influenza (H5N1) outbreak in Asia. During the 2003 SARS outbreak, the Department of State's internal working group, the Department of State-led Interagency Working Group, and the Department of Health and Human Services' (HHS) Emergency Operations Centers kept in constant contact. There were daily phone calls to exchange information, which allowed the Department of State to support, through diplomatic means, HHS and international efforts to gather information and to respond to the epidemic. The Interagency Working Group has addressed international policy and response issues, such as contact tracing and medical evacuations, through a number of meetings since May 2003. The interagency collaboration also allowed the group to address the Avian Influenza outbreak when it was realized to be a major public health issue in January 2004.

The report recommends that the Secretary of Health and Human Services, in consultation with the Secretary of State, work with WHO and official representatives from other WHO member states to strengthen the response capacity of WHO's global infectious disease network. The Department of State is committed, as a foreign policy matter, to work both with WHO and its member states to strengthen the international response to infectious disease outbreaks, and to achieve effective revisions of the International Health Regulations.

The report also recommends authorities for HHS to facilitate contact tracing of arriving passengers determined to be infected with or exposed to SARS. We are pleased to report that the Department of State has been working on those issues in collaboration with our interagency partners since the SARS outbreak. The Department of State has brought together officials of the Departments of Homeland Security and Health and Human Services to facilitate planning and discussion on obtaining passenger contact information. However, as the report notes, serious legal issues still exist for both the United States and for other governments. These center on privacy and access to personal information and may require legislation or regulatory changes. The Department of State will continue to work with its partners to address this issue.

The Department of State also has worked closely with HHS' Centers for Disease Control and Prevention (HHS/CDC) to develop protocols on how to handle medical evacuations of persons suspected or confirmed to have quarantinable diseases, such as SARS. The Department of State's highest priority is the safety and well being of American citizens traveling or residing abroad, including its employees and their families. The Department has direct responsibility for its American employees and their families. Medical evacuation procedures, including how to maintain liaison with HHS/CDC, have been documented, and will shortly be disseminated to our Embassies and consulates throughout the world. It is important to note, however, that capacity for such medical evacuations will always be limited, as will capacity of U.S. medical facilities to handle a large influx of quarantinable patients.

The Department of State believes that this report documents important lessons for other infectious disease outbreaks beyond the 2003 SARS epidemic.

Comments from the World Health Organization

WORLD HEALTH ORGANIZATION ORGANISATION MONDIALE DE LA SANTE

Téléphone Central/Exchange: (+41 22) 791.21.11
Direct: (+41 22) 791.3691
Email:

In reply please refer to: CDS
Prière de rappeler la référence:

Your reference:
Votre référence:

Mr David Gootnick
Director
International Affairs and Trade
US General Accounting Office
Room 4440-C
441 G Street NW
Washington DC 20548
USA

16 April 2004

Dear Mr Gootnick

Thank you for your communication dated 30 March enclosing a draft of the proposed report "Emerging Infectious Diseases: Asian SARS Outbreak Challenged International and National Responses" (GAO-04-564).

We are pleased to enclose our comments on this timely report that provides a detailed insight into the response to SARS within the USA and also in the other affected countries. We particularly welcome the recommendation that the USA should work with representatives of other WHO Member States to "strengthen the response capacity of WHO's global infectious disease network"

Overall the report provides a factual analysis of the events surrounding the emergence of SARS, and in particular addresses the major weaknesses in national and international control efforts in response to the first major disease threat to emerge in the 21st century.

The report presents major criticisms of China, Taiwan and Hong Kong which do not reflect the attitude or response of these areas throughout the SARS response. Certainly there were issues of transparency initially as well as major issues of co-ordination. Certainly their initial responses could be criticized, but they should be credited for the depth and intensity of their control efforts later on. It is of note that there appears to be little emphasis on problematic areas in the response in other countries (e.g. Canada)

There is also some confusion in the document relating to Global Outbreak Alert and Response Network (GOARN) and its relationship to WHO. It is important to note that WHO operates the intelligence, verification and risk assessment mechanism outlined in your report. GOARN can be considered as the operational arm of WHO's response to outbreaks of

cc: Mr D. Hohman, Health Attaché, United States Mission to the United Nations
      Office and other International Organizations at Geneva

ENCLS: As stated

CH-1211 GENEVA 27-SWITZERLAND Fax (+41 22) 791.31.11 http://www.who.int CH-1211 GENEVE 27-SUISSE

Mr David Gootnick, Washington DC   page 2
CDS   16 April 2004

international importance identified. As such, GOARN partners provide assistance in outbreak investigations, specialized laboratory investigation and in the provision of experts to join international response teams.

GOARN is founded on the principle that no one institution has all of the resources and capacities to respond to major multi-country outbreaks like SARS. WHO's strategy for global health security is built on developing networks and partnerships to bring together the resources of technical institutions to respond to all disease outbreaks of international importance

A theme that is reflected a number of times in the report is that WHO was constrained in its response by a lack of resources. Of course, WHO could do with more resources, but WHO's acute response was not constrained by limited resources. WHO managed to support countries throughout the response without launching any external appeals for financial assistance. All requests for assistance from countries for experts and teams were met. However, this did involve significant diversion of internal human and financial resources and it is questionable whether the response could have been sustained for a longer period or that another major event at the same time could have been responded to adequately. That the world is so dependent on a process this fragile and on the personal commitment and sacrifice of WHO and GOARN staff is a concern to us all.

We have placed our more detailed comments in an enclosed document (Annex 1) which address specific points that require correction/clarification. These are taken in order of their appearance in the document.

We trust that you will be able to take these comments on board and we look forward to the publication of this important document in the near future

Yours sincerely,

Dr A. Asamoa-Baah
Assistant Director-General
Communicable Diseases

CH-1211 GENEVA 27-SWITZERLAND Fax (+41 22) 791.31.11 http://www.who.int CH-1211 GENEVE 27-SUISSE

GAO Contacts and Staff Acknowledgments

GAO Contacts

Martin T. Gahart, (202) 512-3596
Cheryl Goodman, (202) 512-6571

Acknowledgments

In addition to the persons named above, Janey Cohen, Patrick Dickriede, Anne Dievler, Suzanne Dove, Sharif Idris, Roseanne Price, Kendall Schaefer, and Richard Seldin made key contributions to this report.

GAO's Mission	The General Accounting Office, the audit, evaluation and investigative arm of Congress, exists to support Congress in meeting its constitutional responsibilities and to help improve the performance and accountability of the federal government for the American people. GAO examines the use of public funds; evaluates federal programs and policies; and provides analyses, recommendations, and other assistance to help Congress make informed oversight, policy, and funding decisions. GAO's commitment to good government is reflected in its core values of accountability, integrity, and reliability.
Obtaining Copies of GAO Reports and Testimony	The fastest and easiest way to obtain copies of GAO documents at no cost is through the Internet. GAO's Web site (www.gao.gov) contains abstracts and full-text files of current reports and testimony and an expanding archive of older products. The Web site features a search engine to help you locate documents using key words and phrases. You can print these documents in their entirety, including charts and other graphics. Each day, GAO issues a list of newly released reports, testimony, and correspondence. GAO posts this list, known as "Today's Reports," on its Web site daily. The list contains links to the full-text document files. To have GAO e-mail this list to you every afternoon, go to www.gao.gov and select "Subscribe to e-mail alerts" under the "Order GAO Products" heading.

Order by Mail or Phone	The first copy of each printed report is free. Additional copies are $2 each. A check or money order should be made out to the Superintendent of Documents. GAO also accepts VISA and Mastercard. Orders for 100 or more copies mailed to a single address are discounted 25 percent. Orders should be sent to:
	
	U.S. General Accounting Office
	441 G Street NW, Room LM
	Washington, D.C. 20548
	
	To order by Phone: Voice: (202) 512-6000
	                           TDD: (202) 512-2537
	                           Fax: (202) 512-6061

To Report Fraud, Waste, and Abuse in Federal Programs	Contact: Web site: www.gao.gov/fraudnet/fraudnet.htm E-mail: fraudnet@gao.gov Automated answering system: (800) 424-5454 or (202) 512-7470
Public Affairs	Jeff Nelligan, Managing Director, NelliganJ@gao.gov (202) 512-4800 U.S. General Accounting Office, 441 G Street NW, Room 7149 Washington, D.C. 20548

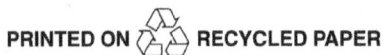

PRINTED ON RECYCLED PAPER

United States
General Accounting Office
Washington, D.C. 20548-0001

Official Business
Penalty for Private Use $300

Address Service Requested